LOUISE TENNEY'S
NUTRITIONAL GUIDE

WITH FOOD COMBINING

Published by
Woodland Books

Notice to the Reader

THIS HEALTH BOOK IS NOT INTENDED TO PRESCRIBE OR DIAGNOSE IN ANY WAY. IT IS NOT MEANT TO BE A SUBSTITUTE FOR PROFESSIONAL HELP. THOSE WHO ARE SICK SHOULD CONSULT THEIR DOCTOR

NEITHER THE AUTHOR NOR THE PUBLISHER DIRECTLY OR INDIRECTLY DISPENSE MEDICAL ADVICE OR PRESCRIBE THE USE OF HERBS, VITAMINS, AND MINERALS AS A FORM OF TREATMENT. THE AUTHOR AND THE PUBLISHER ASSUME NO RESPONSIBILTY IF YOU PRESCRIBE FOR YOURSELF WITHOUT YOUR DOCTOR'S APPROVAL.

Nutritional Guide

©1991 by Louise Tenney, M.H.

Published by

Woodland Health Books

P.O. Box 1422

Provo, Utah 84603

Printed in the United States of America
ISBN 0-913923-79-6

About the Author

Louise Tenney, M.H.

Louise Tenney has dedicated the majority of her adult life to the pursuit, education and teaching of natural approaches to complete health. As an accomplished author and lecturer, Louise has traveled extensively, educating thousands about the importance of individual health. Her speaking assignments have taken her across the United States and Canada, to New Zealand, Brazil and the Caribbean.

Louise has been interested in the nutrition industry all her life, and applies her knowledge to enhance the life of her family and friends. She attended Portland State University where she studied applied chemistry and biology. Louise has studied and researched natural health and herbs intensely for over 15 years, and earned her master herbalist Degree in 1986 from the Emerson College of Herbology in Canada.

Included in Louise Tenney's list of authored works are:

- **Nutritional Guide with Food Combining**
- **Today's Herbal Health**
- **Health Handbook**
- **Modern Day Plagues**
- **Today's Healthy Eating**

Published by Woodland Books

Contents

Introduction

"Men dig their Graves with their own Teeth and die more by those fated Instruments than the Weapons of their Enemies."

Thomas Moffett, 1600 A.D.

Many people eat without thinking about it. They are hungry, so they walk to the refrigerator or cupboard and prepare some food. They halfway chew it, swallow it, and somehow expect it to disappear into their stomachs, to be magically digested and assimilated. Our bodies are wonderful machines, but we often—albeit unknowingly—abuse them. We create stress on the digestive apparatus by eating anything and everything together. A favorite combination of foods for the "fast food connoisseur" is that of a hamburger, french fries and a Coke. Each of these foods is hard to digest to begin with, but the body has the additional burden of trying to separate each one for proper assimilation. The result is often constipation, stomachache and gas. When we are young, we don't realize that these improper eating habits burden the body and gradually inhibit its ability to use the nutrients from our food. The gallbladder, liver, stomach and large and small intestines suffer abuse until we feel the consequences of our decisions.

Health-conscious people shun junk food as much as possible, but some are unaware that there are certain combinations of natural foods which create havoc with digestion and vitality.

This book explains the reasons behind proper food combining and ways to eliminate many digestion difficulties. This new knowledge will reinforce the need for self-discipline and menu planning.

We will examine how correct food combining, proper bowel management, and natural supplements can fortify the body against the ravages of chemicals, pesticides, herbicides, environmental pollution, etc. It will also outline natural approaches to ailments. You can change your life by choosing a healthier lifestyle! This book is dedicated to all those who want to learn for themselves and are willing to apply those principles essential for ideal health.

Louise Tenney, M.H.

Autointoxication

"Hippocrates claimed that chronic disease came from autointoxication, ie., self-poisoning due to constipation. The deposits of accumulated waste in the colon release toxins which inflame the nerves producing rheumatism, neuralgia, melancholia, hysteria, eczema, acne, headaches, and many many other health problems. Hippocrates also taught the way to handle diseases—'Let food be thy medicine.'"

Toxemia and enervation (lowered resistance) are the underlying causes of all diseases. Chronic disease is the "beginning of the end" of slow poisoning caused by toxins in the body. This condition, known as "autointoxication", creates an internal environment where germs and viruses can feed, multiply and flourish. Toxins can be passed on from mother to child before birth, and they can also accumulate from infancy throughout life.

Health experts believe that all sickness begins in the colon. Before World War II, doctors understood this concept and treated illness by giving enemas and colonics. This was before drugs and surgery gained a foothold as the supposed universal antidotes to disease.

Faulty digestion also plays a role in autointoxication. If food is not digested properly, amino acids can be converted by the microbes into powerful toxic substances (phenol, indol, histidine, indican, etc.). These can cause symptoms such as fatigue, nervousness, gastrointestinal upsets, skin problems, headaches, insomnia, glandular and circulatory system disturbances, etc.

Autointoxication also affects the functioning of both liver and brain. It will poison them via the bloodstream and can cause many problems, among them poor memory, personality changes and lower immunity. Autointoxication has also been linked to arthritis, breast disease and emotional disorders. Mental illness can be caused by this condition, especially constipation throughout the intestinal tract.

At the turn of the 20th century, Dr. J. A. Stucky, M.D., made this observation, "That the blood is poisoned through absorption of toxic material from the intestinal canal more frequently than from any other source, I think will not be questioned."

Toxins can result from disturbed body chemistry and are manufactured daily in the intestinal canal and remain in the body. The irritated nerves and poisoned cells protest in the form of rheumatic pains, asthmatic attacks, vertigo, obscure neuroses of eye, ear, nose and throat, neuralgia and headaches.

Medical literature has published reports over the years which support the theory of toxemia and disease.

- One doctor studied over 450 cases of allergies and found that they cleared up when intestinal toxemia was eradicated.

- Another doctor, after observing patients with asthma for 23 years, stated that toxemia is the root cause of the condition and that "the results of treatment justify my position."

- It has been discovered that approximately half of all cases of inflammatory arthritis can be greatly improved by removing the toxins formed in the intestine.

- About one-fourth of all cases of "irregular heartbeats" responded well to elimination of toxemia.

- "Several hundreds of cases" of ear, nose and throat diseases reported in the scientific literature were from autointoxication.

- Toxemia in pregnancy many times stems from being constipated and eating a high-protein diet.

- Many cases of eye diseases and problems were improved when intestinal toxins were removed from the body.

- At an annual meeting of the AMA (American Medical Association) in 1917, a scientific report was shared that stated 517 cases of mental problems were relieved by eradicating intestinal toxemia. These symptoms ranged from mental sluggishness to hallucinations. More recently, schizophrenia has been added to the list of mental disorders which improve when toxemia is eliminated.

Norman W. Walker, D.Sc., Ph.D., has lectured and written extensively about toxemia. In his book, *Colon Health*, he says: "If a person has eaten processed, fried and overcooked foods, devitalized starches, sugar and excessive amounts of salt, his colon cannot possibly be efficient—even if he should have a bowel movement two to three times a day! Instead of furnishing nourishment to the nerves, muscles, cells and tissues of the walls of the colon, such foods can actually cause starvation of the colon."

There is an opening in the cecum (part of the ascending colon) which plays a vital role in colon health. It is called the "ileocecal valve". The physiology text, Guyton, says: "A principal function of the ileocecal valve is to prevent back flow of fecal contents from the colon into the small intestine. Usually the valve can resist reverse pressure of as much as 50-60 centimeters of water." Health author Dr. William F. Welles explains that, "This means the valve is designed to resist considerable pressure before it lets fecal contents re-enter the small intestine ... It is clear from this that the ileocecal valve is incompetent in the majority of

Americans. As the ileocecal valve becomes incompetent, the contents of the large bowel back up into the no longer sterile environment of the small intestine, toxins enter the bloodstream, the liver becomes overburdened, and not only high cholesterol, but also autointoxication result."

PROPER ELIMINATION

The five organs of elimination are: the bowel, the kidneys, the lungs, the liver and the skin. The skin? Yes! It is often referred to as "the third kidney".

In hot weather we drink more water and perspire through the skin more profusely. During cold weather we seem to drink fewer liquids and perspire less. Then we eliminate mainly through urination. When the skin is clogged by dead cells, soap accumulations and other matter, it cannot "breathe" properly. It is prevented from discharging toxins out of the body. This important eliminative channel can suffocate and trap waste materials, which otherwise would cleanse out through the pores. It is suggested by health experts that a daily "dry skin massage" is beneficial for this problem. Dr. Bernard Jensen, in his book "Beyond Basic Health" says: "Brush for above five minutes before showering or taking a bath in the morning. Brushing the skin removes the uric acid crystals, catarrh, and other acid wastes that come up through the pores of the skin. I recommend this as 'dry bathing'. You can do it twice a day, if you desire."

"We build new skin every day, and brushing the skin twice daily helps the body to eliminate, get rid of old skin cells, and keep pores open. Some patients told me they had begun to perspire again after skin brushing, when they hadn't been perspiring for years."

The keys to proper elimination through the five organs are daily exercise, proper diet (including herbs and supplements), positive mental attitude and stress control.

Constipation results when the bowels are sluggish and the peristaltic movements do not function well.

HOW TO GO ON A CLEANSE

The human body was designed to operate at a very high level of health. However, due to the interference of various elements; i.e.: faulty eating habits, emotional and physical stresses, environmental pollutants and daily intake of refined foods; this is not always possible. The body will try to compensate for the imbalance created by these factors. It will adjust and adapt as much as possible, until all avenues are exhausted and it succumbs to weakness and disease.

To restore health, you must first CLEANSE, then BUILD. The body will not readily accept the health-building properties of juices, fresh fruits and vegetables or herbs if it is filled with toxins and mucus. Therefore, it is important to clean the body of these barriers. We then strengthen the body with the vitamins, minerals, herbs, enzymes, amino acids, etc., found in these natural foods. The result is increased vitality, energy and zest for life. However, you do not have to wait until disease strikes to go on a cleanse. Everyone accumulates toxins throughout the years, and it is good to embark upon a periodic and thorough 'housecleaning.'

It is recommended that a person go on a "juice fast" anywhere from twenty-four hours to four days. To facilitate cleansing, an herbal enema is suggested.

The following herbs Cleanse the Body: Red clover; chaparral; echinacea; pau d'arco (taheebo); cascara sagrada; black walnut; golden seal; burdock; devil's claw; fenugreek; gentian; oregon grape and psyllium.

During the fasting period fresh juices and homemade soups can be taken. The abundance of nutrients in the above will assist in the detoxification of the body. Avoid using fluoridated water, and aluminum pans and cooking utensils at all costs. During the first part of the fast you may notice that you experience flu-like symptoms or maybe even skin rashes or blemishes. Don't worry, because this is nature's way of telling you that the toxins are being released. It is a good sign, and it will pass.

Suggested Juices: Beet; Carrot; Cabbage; Cucumber; Celery; Apple. All of these should be freshly juiced.

Beet Juice: Beets are blood builders. The nutrients also nourish the lymphatic system, kidneys and bladder. Beets contain vitamins A, C, B complex, iron, calcium, potassium, phosphorus and sodium.

Carrot Juice: This is very helpful for cleansing and nourishing. Less than a full cup of this fresh juice contains more than 30,000 units of vitamin A and an abundance of calcium. It assists in restoring balance within the intestinal tract.

Cabbage Juice: Cabbage is healing to the stomach tissues and helps encourage the appetite. Cabbage provides sulphur, calcium, iodine and vitamin U, which helps alleviate ulcers.

Cucumber Juice: Cucumbers contain silicon, calcium, potassium, sulphur, and vitamins B, B1, B2 and helps equalize blood pressure.

Celery Juice: Celery juice helps clear the body of mucus. Celery's high calcium content feeds the nerves and alleviates insomnia. It is rich in natural sodium. This assists digestion and mobility of joints and tendons.

Apple Juice: The malic acid and glucose in apple juice are excellent for the nerves. It purifies the blood and helps regenerate health, purify the skin, and other tissues. Apple juice provides vitamins A, B complex and C. It also contains high amounts of potassium.

PROGRAM

(Modify this program to fit your needs. A weak person should only fast for one day; stronger individuals may fast from 3 days to a week. If a person is really weak, he or she should not fast at all, because the body's energy is so depleted).

1. Upon arising, drink one glass of warm, pure water with the added juice of one half lemon. Throughout the day use other juices or pure water, as you become thirsty.

2. In the afternoon or evening, twice a week, use an herbal enema.

3. Take a brisk walk once a day, for one half hour.

4. Try to forget your worries and stresses.

*Dr. Norman W. Walker, authority on juice fasting, recommends that the safest way to fast is to take fruit juices only for three to four days at a time, and then drink vegetable juices and eat raw vegetables and fruits for two to three days afterward.

Acute Diseases
(Colds, flu and fever)

"Disease is a warning. It is a friend, not a foe, of mankind. It manifests itself in its various forms, from a slight cold to the more severe inflammations, for the sole purpose of ridding the body of accumulated poisons."

Dr. Wager, The Law of Disease

Nature provides a built-in cleansing mechanism, which is sometimes misinterpreted as a negative symptom because it manifests itself in the form of an acute disease. Dr. Henry Lindlahr, (a medical doctor in the early 1900s), was considered an expert on this subject. His works constantly ring of logic and truth. His fundamental laws of cure, which form the basic principles of the science of natural healing, show that acute disease itself is a cure. It represents Nature's efforts to purify and regenerate the system.

What is an acute disease? Acute diseases have a rapid onset and run a short course and a short period of distress and discomfort, as compared to chronic disease. Chronic disease has a slow onset and lasts for a long period of time.

Common Acute Diseases: Appendicitis, Asthma (Acute), Bladder infections, Boils, Bright's disease, Bronchitis, Chicken pox, Colds, Congestion of the kidneys, Coughs, Croup, Cystitis, Diarrhea, Diphtheria, Dysentery, Ear infections, Endocarditis (Acute), Enteritis (Acute), Eye infections, Gastritis, German measles, Glaucoma, Gout (Acute), Gonorrhea, Hayfever, Hemorrhages, Hives, Hydrophobia, Influenza, Jaundice, Laryngitis, Lung problems, Mumps, Nephritis (Acute), Phlebitis, Pleurisy, Pneumonia, Scarlet fever, Syphilis, Smallpox, Tetanus (lock jaw), Tonsilitis, Toothache, Typhoid fever, Tuberculosis, Whopping cough, Yellow fever.

Colds, flu and fevers are a natural eliminative process ... a safety valve which the body opens of its own accord to give it a chance to eradicate toxins. A short fast will help hasten the stage of acute disease. Use lemon, lime, grapefruit and orange juices diluted with pure water; also herbal teas. No sweet juices such as grape or apple should be used during an acute disease, as they cause fermentation in the intestinal tract. Acute disease is a healing and cleansing of the body, so the body is really trying to eliminate from the cells and organs the accumulated toxins and poisons. It brings them to the stomach to be eliminated. Cleansing is stopped when you eat food because the body has to use its energy to digest it. People usually feel better when this natural cleanse is stopped because their "aches" and "pains" go away for awhile. Eating, however, will stop this vital process and will drive the mucus and toxins deeper into the body, where it will take a greater cleanse next time to get rid of it. Eating will deplete the body of energy to heal. Why do people 'catch colds' after they are chilled? Dr. Lindlahr explains: "Taking cold may be caused by chilling the surface of the body or part of the body. In the chilled portions of the skin the pores close; the blood recedes into the interior, and as a result, the elimination of poisonous gases and exudates is locally suppressed. This 'catching cold' through being exposed to a cold draft, through wet clothing, etc., is not necessarily followed by more serious consequences. If the system is not much encumbered with morbid matter and if the kidneys and intestines are in fairly good working order, these organs will assist the temporarily inactive skin to take care of the extra amount of waste and morbid materials and eliminate them without difficulty. The greater the vitality and the more normal the composition of the blood, the more effectively the system as a whole will react in such an emergency and throw off the morbid materials which were not eliminated through the skin."

Dr. Lindlahr taught and proved in his medical practice that all acute diseases are the same in nature and purpose and that they run the same course through five stages of inflammation. These stages are: INCUBATION, AGGRAVATION, DESTRUCTION, ABATEMENT and RECONSTRUCTION. All five stages are necessary for complete cleansing and subsequent healing of the body. Every disease, whether it is acute or chronic, has to go through five stages of inflammation. This is a natural law of nature.

Some people think that they are healthy because they never get 'sick.' Yet they have improper diets and allow stress to bind them up. These people need to initiate a cleanse by going on the same program as those who come down with the acute diseases. Persons who eat devitalized foods and who go year after year without a 'housecleaning' may find themselves someday with a fullblown chronic disease, and wonder where it came from.

I & II. INCUBATION AND AGGRAVATION: These stages are when there is toxic material in the body, trying to eliminate through an acute disease. The energy and nutrients of the body are depleted from stress, personal problems and life, and bad eating habits. The body is unable to eliminate toxins, poisons, drugs, etc., and they accumulate in the tissues, causing an obstruction at some point. This period may last from a few hours to several days, weeks, months or even years. During this stage, waste matter, poisons, air pollution, germs, parasites and other uninvited guests congregate in certain parts and organs of the body. When they have accumulated to such an extent as to interfere with the normal functions of life or to endanger the health and life of the body, the life forces begin to react to the obstruction or threatening danger by creating the inflammatory process. The body is unable to resist and does not have the energy or power to overcome the natural attraction to germs. Vitality reserve is low, and has been all used up. If the toxins and mucus are not eliminated, they are thrown further into the organs of the body and will build up in the joints, the organs, the lymphatic system and around the heart and veins and start to solidify for chronic conditions of the body. The tonsils and appendix protect the body and help in the eliminating process in acute diseases. If they have been surgically removed, then the body has to work harder to get rid of waste matter and toxins, through the lymphatics and liver. If cleansing is suppressed at this stage (through eating or taking drugs), then mucus, toxins and pus will harden in the body for chronic conditions of the organs.

III. DESTRUCTION STAGE: This is the stage where the battle between the immune system and the toxins of disease gradually progress, accompanied by a corresponding increase of fever and inflamed tissues where they can incubate into chronic conditions. This is the stage where there is a lot of pus and mucus in the body, when tissues are being broken down. The organs at this stage are holding pus, mucus, and toxins and retaining them in the organs. When the body is suppressed by drugs and eating, the toxins stay in the organs and cause pneumonia, tuberculosis, infantile paralysis, spinal meningitis, asthma, emphysema, bronchitis and many other diseases. Using natural methods will assist nature in eliminating toxins without causing serious damage.

IV. ABATEMENT STAGE: This is the stage where excess waste begins to eliminate. The body is now strong enough to win the battle. Appropriate treatment will build up the blood, increase the vitality and promote natural elimination. Then the poisons and germs of disease will be overcome and eliminated. The glands in the system are absorbing all the excess waste as in the lymphatic glands and the intestinal glands. The fever reduces, and the symptoms decrease. As they are being absorbed and with the right treatment, the body will expel the toxins. If the cleansing is suppressed at this stage, the glands will become congested. This will result in lymphatic congestion, glandular secretions, tumors, cysts, moles and skin diseases. This stage sets the environment for all diseases.

V. RECONSTRUCTION STAGE: When the period of absorption has run its course and the affected areas have been cleared of the morbid accumulations and obstructions, then during the fifth stage of inflammation the work of rebuilding begins. The struggle has been more or less destructive to the cells, tissues, blood vessels and organs of the areas involved. They must now be reconstructed, and this last stage of inflammatory process is, therefore, in a way the most important. This is the process of regeneration of the injured parts of the body. If the process of reconstruction is interfered with or interrupted before it is complete, the microzyma will continue to create germs of putrefaction and the affected parts and organs will not have a chance to become entirely clean, well or strong. The body will remain in an abnormal, diseased condition and its functional activity will be seriously handicapped. The body is still weak at this stage and has a lot of poisons. This is the building stage, and if it is suppressed at this time, the absorption glands remain full. They swell up, then they shrink and cannot produce the hormones properly. Now we have low hormone output, low lymphatic absorption, and the intestinal tract is still coated. We experience indigestion, anemia and deficiencies in the body, and an imbalance is created. We cannot absorb our nutrients properly. We have suppressed an acute disease at the stage where we should be restoring the cells with the proper environment for chronic disease, and now we are told they are incurable diseases. The diseases we are treating now are: AIDS, leukemia, all kinds of cancer, candida, diabetes, herpes, Epstein-Barr, etc.

When treating acute diseases with natural methods—such as cleaning the bowels, fasting (stop eating), citrus juices and herbal teas, water therapy, fresh air, rest and some physical manipulation—it will always be best if the five stages are allowed to run their natural course.

Dr. Lindlahr maintained that natural remedies can be applied from the first sign of an acute disease, at the slightest manifestation of inflammatory and fever symptoms.

One of the principles that he stressed is that prevention is better than the cure. Orthodox medical science has learned that this is true as far as surroundings are concerned, but has not yet applied this principal to internal conditions. The theory espoused by modern medical science is to 'kill the germ and cure the disease.' With the drugs they prescribe they have developed drug therapies that suppress the acute disease. This complicates the condition and/or throws it deeper into the organs to cause a chronic disease later.

The first temporary violent effect of poisonous drugs, in active doses, is usually due to Nature's effort to overcome and eliminate these substances. Continued use of drugs often results in complete exhaustion and paralysis of mental and physical powers. Each drug breeds new disease symptoms, which are in their turn, "cured" by other poisons until the body is too weak to throw off the toxins and drugs.

If we use drugs or food, they will suppress the flu or cold, and that which should have been eliminated will be retained within the body. As long as we continue to suppress the natural process of elimination, the toxic material will begin to settle in the organs of the body to eventually create what we call chronic disease ... such as arthritis, diabetes, chronic asthma, etc.

We must emphasize that you can eat a highly nutritious diet and still create a toxic condition in your body. How is that? Well, if you allow negative emotions to breed inside and take root, this will affect the function of your body. The stress will upset your organs and glands and will turn the food you ingest into toxic substances. Hate, especially, is such a strong emotion that it will wreak havoc and turmoil inside of you by producing toxic acids. It will jeopardize your immune system. You can see what stress can do to you if you are in a weakened condition. If junk food is consumed, with no regard to healthful eating habits or supplements, then the body cannot become fortified to handle stress. We must learn to cultivate a positive attitude, as well as discipline ourselves to eat foods with high-nutrient density. We cannot avoid lifestyle changes and stresses, but we can strengthen our immune systems. Proper bowel management, cleansing and a positive mental attitude can con ribute to a longer, healthier life.

Metal Poisoning:
A Health Hazard

TOXIC METALS

Toxic metals are systemic poisons which inhibit biochemical enzyme functioning and which can cause fatigue from body malfunction. These toxic metals are non-essential trace metals and are known to accumulate in tissues and biological fluids, producing acute and chronic toxicity.

Depression and suicidal thoughts seem to be a natural part of heavy metal poisoning. Mental depression has a sudden onset and usually is not caused by any one set of circumstances. It seems to arrive when everything is going great. Doctors (after putting their depressed patients through numerous tests) finally refer them to a psychiatrist, which only prolongs their misery. This can make them feel guilty for the feeling they can't control.

Common toxic metals are aluminum, arsenic, cadmium, lead, mercury and nickel. Nickel is widely used as a catalyst to harden fats. It is found in most margarines, commercial peanut butter and hardened shortenings. It is in drinking water, refined and processed foods, superphosphate fertilizers and tobacco smoke.

ALUMINUM

Aluminum contamination is a major health threat today. High levels are showing up in the human body. Absorption of aluminum by the body is not only associated with Alzheimer's Disease, but with Parkinson's disease and dialysis dementia. It also lowers the body's immune system. Pots and pans, foil, antacids and baking powder are common items with aluminum. It is found in pickles, relishes and some cheeses, in soft drinks and beers in uncoated aluminum cans. It is also found in water supplies and the soil. Aluminum inhibits fluorine and phosphorus metabolism, resulting over a long period of time in a loss of essential minerals from the bones and sets the stage for osteoporosis. The Harvard Medical School Newsletter published an article that stated that America is experiencing an epidemic of osteoporosis in the elderly and by the age of thirty-five the seed is sown.

ARSENIC

Arsenic is in our environment as a by-product of industry. It's in the air, a pollutant that we are exposed to each day of our lives. It is not only in the air, but found in the refining processes of glass making, pesticide plants spray, and in coal fired boilers. It is found in hidden items such as dishwasher sealant and has been known to poison whole families. Arsenic is in coal and in the air wherever it is burned. Coal workers are at potential risk. There is also an accumulation of arsenic from liquor.

Arsenic settles in the muscles and back. Spasms in the back can pull the spine out of place. Arsenic poisoning produces nervous irritations in various parts of the body. It is found mainly in the liver. In females arsenic levels increase in the blood during menstruation and during the fifth and sixth months of pregnancy. Symptoms of arsenic toxicity are fatigue, loss of pain sensation and inflammation of the lining membrane of the stomach and intestines (Gastroenteritis). Arsenic replaces essential trace minerals, which disrupts the body's metabolism.

CADMIUM

Cadmium is a by-product of industry and is extremely widespread. It is in the air, soil and water. It is used as a hardener in tires. We acquire it by absorbing it through our tissues. People with hypertension usually have elevated cadmium levels and are usually low in zinc. It affects the pancreas and spleen. Coronary artery disease tends to rise when the intake of cadmium is high. It is also found in bone marrow and in the male testes.

Cadmium can produce high blood pressure, kidney and liver damage, anemia and a host of other symptoms as well as fatigue. Over many years scientists used to think that nothing could remove cadmium deposits. Science has proven that iron and vitamin C together can reduce cadmium. Selenium and zinc are the best protection against cadmium toxicity. Don't let anyone tell you that minerals are not vital in our world today.

LEAD

Lead poisoning, as we have mentioned before, is a major pollutant in our environment and we breath it constantly. It is a frightening health threat to our children. Lead causes a gradual build-up of chronic problems, such as allergies. It also decreases immunity to diseases. It accumulates in the tissues. Low levels can bring subtle changes and problems. It is felt that most people in the United States may be suffering partial brain dysfunction as a result of lead pollution. Lead intake increases twenty-five percent when you smoke.

Lead deposits in the brain and causes brain damage, retardation, and hyperactivity. Many children are born with high levels of lead and cadmium, which causes nervous disorders similar to epileptic-type nerve transmission problems. When lead goes into the brain, it displaces copper, iron and zinc. Oxygen is essential to proper brain function, and the lack of copper in the brain causes the cells to "breathe" with difficulty. Zinc deficiency can cause learning and memory difficulties.

Lead interferes with the normal activities of the nervous system and causes damage to the myelin sheath (a fat-like substance forming the principal component in the brain and the covering over the nerves).

Lead interferes with the energy in the body, with enzyme exchange, as well as the nervous system. It accumulates in the bones and displaces calcium. It causes the body to be more susceptible to diseases, muscle weakness, tremors, gout, lack of coordination, clumsiness, and symptoms similar to multiple sclerosis.

Lead by-products are found in auto exhaust, air pollution, canned food and canned drinks, mascara, pewter tableware, plumbing, roadside vegetables, tobacco smoke, water, wine, some hair colorings and ceramic glaze. Lead activates the enzyme hyaluronidase, which breaks down the synovial fluid in bone joints.

It also contributes to the deterioration of tissue and collagen and makes you more susceptible to diseases like cancer and arthritis.

MERCURY

The amalgam used to fill teeth is 40 to 50 percent mercury. Under the pressure of hard chewing, mercury vapor is released from the fillings, and is absorbed by the body. To make matters worse, the bacteria in the mouth (the same strain blamed for plaque), can convert mercury into methyl mercury, the most toxic form. It is not only toxic, but has an affinity for proteins, attaching itself to blood cells and interfering with the function of the glands, nervous system and the brain. It has a potentially dangerous effect on the lungs, heart, liver and kidneys.

It depresses the immune system. Dr. Carlton Fredericks said that mercury toxicity could have been responsible for some of his patients' susceptibility to yeast infections and allergies.

Mercury is found in treated seeds for farm planting, cosmetics, fabric softeners, fish and sea foods, fungicides, laxatives containing calomes, and some hemorrhoidal suppository preparations.

Mercury causes depression, irritability, tremors, dizziness and diarrhea. As the metal builds up over a period of years, it leads to progressive degeneration of the brain, liver, kidneys and intestines.

NICKEL

Nickel settles in the sinuses, head, heart or spinal column. It acts as a poison to the nervous system. Too much nickel in the human body may paralyze the spinal column. Many locked joints are caused by an accumulation of nickel. It is cancer-causing, and respiratory cancer has been known to develop within three years of inhaling nickel-contaminated dust.

Nickel carbonyl is found in cigarette smoke and is harmful to both the smoker and non-smoker who breathe "second-hand" cigarette smoke pollution.

PROTECTION AGAINST TOXIC METALS

Vitamin A is necessary for the cells to be able to eliminate the toxic metal absorbed from chemicals in food, air and water.

Vitamin B-complex protects the immune system. Under stress the B vitamins need to be increased. They protect the nerve sheath, and prevents lead from damaging the nervous system.

Vitamin C with bioflavonoids stimulates natural interferon production in the body. Interferon protects and strengthens the immune system. Vitamin C is essential to take each day to keep our tissues saturated and protect the body from toxic metals. Bioflavonoids increase the strength of the capillary walls, reduces inflammation and helps keep the collagen healthy. Collagen is a cement that sticks the cells together and is essential for healthy muscles, skin and joints.

Fiber dilutes stool bile acids and reduces the concentration of toxic carcinogenic substances in the colon and eliminates them. Fiber also eliminates excess fat in the body. Fiber such as psyllium, oat bran and whole grains are excellent. Apple pectin removes lead. It is changed into galacturonic acid (one of natures cleansing agents) after digestion. This acid combines with lead to form an insoluble metallic salt that cannot be absorbed. Eat fiber daily.

Oral Chelation is a formula with vitamins, minerals, glandulars, amino acids and herbs used to clean the system. Natural nutrients that gradually dissolve and eliminate deposits on the arteries. It is very effective to rid the body of high levels of toxic metals.

Distilled Water is a natural chelation, always use with minerals.

Lecithin combines with choline and produces acetylcholine, a vital neurotransmitter. Lecithin is an essential brain food.

Calcium is an indispensable mineral; it actually penetrates the bones and slowly displaces lead. It prevents accumulation of lead from the intestinal tract. The best calcium is an herbal calcium formula.

Germanium binds with toxic metals to prevent them from being dispersed throughout the body. It improves stamina and endurance. It increases the body's production of interferon which stops the multiplication of viruses.

Garlic is a natural antibiotic, lowers blood pressure, and cleans the veins, it helps in digestion and is excellent for lungs and respiratory problems. Garlic is rich in sulphur, which attracts metals and eliminates them from the body. Garlic contains germanium and selenium with chelation ability to neutralize heavy metal toxicity.

Ginkgo is a strong antioxidant, and free-radical scavenger, and increases the flow of nutrients and oxygen to all cells. It improves memory, mental efficiency and concentration. Reduces anxiety, tension, symptoms of senility and age related cerebral disorders.

Gotu Kola is food for the brain. Purifies the blood and helps eliminate fatigue and memory loss. Increases mental alertness. It is a tonic for the whole body. Helps rebuild energy reserves, especially after a nervous breakdown. Protects the body against toxins.

Herbs containing sulphur are excellent to protect the body from heavy metal toxicity. Horseradish, watercress, alfalfa, burdock, dandelion, comfrey, garlic, onions, sarsaparilla, kelp, echinacea, lobelia, mullein, parsley, cayenne, chaparral, eyebright, nettle and fennel.

Zinc is an essential mineral and helps to eliminate lead from the body as well as other toxins.

Kelp attacks itself to any lead that is present and carries it harmlessly out of the system.

Co-Q 10 protects the immune system. Strengthens the body's resistance to stress and disease by making tissues stronger and healthier. Aids in oxygenation within the cells and tissues. Good for heart disease, aging, cancer and obesity.

Chlorophyll is nature's natural cleanser. Cleans the blood stream and eliminates toxins from the bowels.

Suma contains germanium to protect the immune system. Protects the body from stress. Improves circulation, heart and arthritis. It also balances hormones.

Algin is a natural extract from kelp. It is a concentrated form of nutrient that is found very effective in eliminating the body of radioactive strontium 90. It is also beneficial to eliminate the chemical additives that we ingest daily.

Algin grabs hold of the toxic material and excretes it out of the body. It acts like a magnet, drawing the radioactive material and other unwanted toxic waste that is harmful to the system.

Nervine herbs are essential to protect the central nervous system and the brain. They feed and nourish these nerves. Hops, lady's slipper, scullcap, valerian, passion flower, wood betony, chamomile, black cohosh and lobelia.

Hydrochloric acid and digestive enzymes are essential nutrients, such as minerals that bind metals and eliminate them from the body.

Heavy metals create negative electrical current and creates an imbalance in the body, as well as other numerous problems.

Selenium rids the body of lead, cadmium, mercury, herbicides, pesticides and drugs.

Proper Digestion

The body will take marvelous care of the food you eat through the process of digestion. We often eat hastily, thus cheating ourselves out of digestion's many health benefits.

What happens to our food after it enters the mouth? We don't really think about it ... we either chew or gulp and it's gone! There is a specific coordination of activities within the four parts of the body involved with digestion. These areas are: the mouth and esophagus, stomach, small intestine and large intestine.

THE MOUTH AND ESOPHAGUS

1. You smell the wonderful aroma and your mouth starts "watering".

2. You taste the food and your saliva REALLY starts to flow.

3. You chew the food slowly and carefully. This will allow the saliva to mix well and start this intricate breakdown with an enzyme produced by the salivary glands. It is called pytalin. The more thoroughly your body digests food, the better it will assimilate the nutrients from it. Food is meant to be enjoyed ... (in moderation, of course), so why not taste it longer? Also, if you don't swallow large chunks of food, you will eat less. It then travels to that adaptable pouch, your stomach.

4. Medications such as antihistamines and diuretics tend to dry the mucus membranes and therefore interfere with the secretion of the enzyme amylase (pepsin). This can alter the initial function of digestion and when the food enters the stomach digestion is already incomplete. This creates chronic gas and bloating. In this case it is the lack of hydrochloric acid that is the problem. This deficiency should not be blamed because of improper chewing.

THE IMPORTANCE OF CHEWING WELL

Good chewing is vital for a strong immune system, digestive system and colon health. Any disease can be improved when chewing is practiced in earnest. The healing process is speeded up when proper chewing is used in practice.

Health depends on nutrition, and nutrition comes from the food we eat. By chewing very well, many troubles can be resolved. You will have clearer thinking, more energy, and toxins will not build up as quickly.

Why is chewing important? Solid foods cannot be broken down properly in the stomach without proper chewing. Foods must be mixed with saliva. Saliva contains the digestive enzyme ptyalin, which changes complex carbohydrates into simple sugar, which in turn, converts to glucose. If we do not chew well, the ptyalin enzyme cannot permeate the grains and the starch does not change into glucose. The stomach has no digestive juices which will simplify carbohydrates; this is where fermentation takes place if foods are not prepared by chewing. The result is excessive gas and discomfort in the stomach.

Chewing stimulates the stomach, intestines, and all the digestive organs. The liver sends more bile to the duodenum. Concentrating on chewing will also relax your nervous system.

Saliva increases with chewing. There are three pairs of salivary glands. The parotid glands are located under the ears on both sides of the head. They are much larger than the other glands and produce the greatest amount of saliva. The molars help to stimulate the parotid glands to produce a ptyalin-rich saliva. Salty and bitter foods also stimulate these glands. The submaxillary glands are located along the side of the lower jawbone. They produce additional saliva needed for sour and oily foods, and for chewing meat. The sublingual glands are smaller, and are found at the floor of the mouth. When we eat sweet foods or bite into fruits and vegetables, these glands produce a thinner saliva to dilute strong sweet tastes.

The true taste of food is in the end taste. Each bite should be chewed 32 times. To obtain the real benefit of grains, proper chewing is vital. Through the careful practice of chewing, you will be able to distinguish and enjoy the following three tastes: beginning taste, middle taste and end taste.

Chewing food properly helps our taste return to natural foods. Fast eating destroys our ability to taste properly and enjoy natural foods. Chewing slowly also protects us from poisons, or toxic materials, by warning us by strange tastes.

Chewing helps us control our appetite. When we chew well, the stomach feels full when it is at 80-90 percent of its capacity. To lose weight, chew three times as much.

The stomach is the seat of most diseases. When we overeat, swallow big pieces of food, use strong spices, eat too much sugar or salt, drink alcohol, coffee, very hot soup or tea; or eat in the middle of the night we are indulging in improper eating habits. When we eat without chewing well, large pieces of food remain in the stomach for a long time and the stomach excretes more acid and creates fermentation—with its accompanying gas, burps, and belches. Then real stomach problems can begin.

Chewing helps strengthen the teeth and gums. The saliva excretes a special hormone for maintaining strong teeth. This hormone, called parotin, is only produced by the parotid glands through chewing. It is absorbed by the lymph vessels through the mouth during chewing, and then it goes into the bloodstream. This unique hormone stimulates cell metabolism and thus renews the entire body.

The greatest benefit of all that chewing provides is increasing T-cell function. One of the special jobs of the hormone parotin is to stimulate the thymus gland, thereby producing more T-cells. This has a vital function in the immune system.

THE STOMACH

The stomach weighs approximately four and a half ounces and an adult male can put five to eight pints into it (except for holidays and special occasions). It consists of "folds" which expand as food is introduced. Some people try to stuff as much as they can into it out of habit. It is best to stop eating before you are completely full. It takes more energy to digest food than for any other bodily function. Therefore, the more food there is to take care of, the less energetic you will feel. Proteins and fats take longer to digest than grains, fruits or vegetables. If you don't want to fall asleep, eat lightly!

The digestion of carbohydrates starts in the mouth; the acid environment of the stomach stops this process until the duodenum provides an alkaline medium. If the stomach has not produced enough HCL the pancreas will not be triggered to produce the bicarbonate ions. The lack of HCL secretion in the stomach will influence the digestion of carbohydrates and fats, as well as protein. When the food enters the stomach it produces four major digestive aids: mucous, acid, pepsin and gastrin (a hormone). In the stomach hydrochloric acid is responsible for breaking down the food, destroying germs and utilizing the pepsin (a protein-digesting enzyme). Too much hydrochloric acid causes stomach ulcers and too little will increase the chances of developing gastric cancer.

Excess hydrochloric acid is produced by anger, worry and anxiety, which causes the stomach walls to become swollen and inflamed. Emotions play a major-part and changes can be affected by resentment, depression, and disgusted and fearful attitudes.

Emotional stress plays a major role in stomach digestive disorders. The stomach is a very sensitive organ and nervous problems can slow down or speed up digestion. Under acute stress the stomach has a tendency to shut off acid production. Chronic stress causes an excessive excretion of hydrochloric acid, which can cause acid indigestion. This irritation of the mucous membrane lining of the stomach is what causes ulcers and hiatal hernia (regurgitation reflex in the esophagus). It is a big mistake to eat while in this state of emotional stress. Only natural food should be eaten to create cooperation between the acid and buffer for proper digestion.

SMALL INTESTINE

The next step in digestion after the stomach does its churning is into the duodenal areas of the small intestine. This is where the food comes in contact with enzymes from the pancreas and bile system.

The pancreas secretes enzymes for the digestion of carbohydrates, fats and protein, as well as breaks down nucleic acids RNA and DNA. This is where the buffer bicarbonate secretion is created in this colon area which, if it is sufficient, will neutralize the hydrochloric acid as it enters the small intestine from the stomach. This is where duodenal ulcers are created if there is not enough bicarbonate to act as a neutralizer.

The small intestine is the most important organ in proper digestion. This is where we absorb most of our nutrients. The mixing of water, salt, mucous and numerous enzymes are completed combined for absorption.

The small intestine is so important that its loss would demand intravenous feeding. As long as we keep our small intestine in proper order we continue to acquire nourishment to sustain life.

GALL BLADDER AND LIVER

The next important organs to help with digestion are the gall bladder and the liver, which secrete a substance called bile. This bile acts as a detergent to emit bicarbonate, which makes solubles out of fats and helps neutralize the hydrochloric acid. The bile salts also stimulate the removal of organize waste products and various trace minerals throughout the body. This is the part of the body where fat-soluble vitamins A, D, E, and K are digested. Bile also promotes the normal peristaltic action of the colon. Constipation can occur if the gall bladder is not functioning properly.

The concentrated bile from the gall bladder is stored between meals, then when meals are eaten the stored bile is released by contractions of that organ. If you don't have your gall bladder anymore, you can develop bloating and also become deficient in vitamin A, D, E, and K. You also have a constant dripping of bile from the liver all day long, and when meal times arrive there is not enough to digest the food properly. The constant drip irritates the small intestine which can cause colitis. If the gall bladder has been removed it would be beneficial to drink a lot of water throughout the day and this will help dilute the constant drip of bile.

LARGE INTESTINE

When digestion is not functioning properly the large intestine can be in trouble. If there has been faulty peristaltic action causing constipation, this will cause diverticulosis, putting fermented material in the pockets of the colon which causes problems. This is where most of our health problems stem from.

The rectum is the last link in the digestive system. This is where irritations, itching and hemorrhoids can develop. When a person becomes ill it slows the transit time of food. An enema or herbal laxative should be used to clean out the system.

DIGESTION DISTURBANCES

BLOATING: This can also be due to liver and gall bladder sluggishness. Add lecithin, inositol, choline, and methionine (an amino acid), and B6.

DIGESTION OF FOOD: Dr. W. A. Hemmings, an English allergist, feels that poor digestion of food can lead to the absorption of partially-digested food, which may in turn induce allergic reactions.

FLATULENCE: This is increased when starting on a health diet and introducing too much new food at first, such as nuts, beans, cereals and other new foods. This is caused from the metabolizing of fiber content in these new foods by gas-producing bacteria in the colon. As your body becomes used to these new foods it will produce its own enzymes to help the gas problems. Always introduce new foods one at a time and in small amounts.

WEIGHT PROBLEMS: A poor digestive system can cause obesity. When we do not completely digest certain fats and proteins they can be stored as body fat. When the body does not obtain what it needs it constantly tries to obtain it by creating a never-ending appetite. A vicious cycle ensues until the body is satisfied with enough nutrients.

MALABSORPTION

When the body is unable to absorb and metabolize nutrients from foods, it is called "malabsorption". People whose bodies are not balanced and who do not digest their foods properly may not be obtaining adequate nutrition. They may experience fatigue, irritability, moodiness, and may complain of being unable to gain or lose weight. Both obese and underweight individuals need to evaluate their digestion, to see if that is the problem. Stress, glandular imbalance and parasites may also play a role in these disorders. Proper food combining allows the digestive system to concentrate on one or two foods at a time and promotes balance in that system. Eating on a regular schedule and avoiding in-between-meal snacking are other ways to assist better digestive function.

The type of food a person eats can also alter their psychological outlook on life. Milk and sugar products provoke negative reactions in many people. Milk has been known to cause depression, weepiness, and feelings of helplessness and the inability to cope with everyday problems. Sugar can aggravate emotions such as despair, depression and alienation from others. Many times these symptoms can be linked to allergic reactions to these foods. Even wheat has caused emotional disorders. It is theorized that the use of pesticides and chemical fertilizers used on wheat today could be part of the reason.

Overgrowth of the yeast organism, Candida albicans, is a common plague today. It can play a part in immune dysfunction, allergies, and even mental instability. Karen relates a problem she had with Candida. She experienced psychological and emotional "low times", and at one time even considered suicide. She yelled at her kids, didn't want her husband to come around her, and she "caught every disease that came along". Her children were all born with thrush, which is caused by Candida. Karen didn't know what to do. She seemed to always be sick, emotionally and physically. Then one day she read an article on natural health. She went to the health food store and bought books on nutrition. She changed her diet and eliminated refined foods, and exchanged them for whole foods. She still experienced indigestion and gas, however, until she began taking digestive herbs and eliminating meat from her diet. Karen finally found relief by taking acidophilus, which helped with the yeast. She also took vitamins, minerals, grains, raw seeds and nuts, and raw fruits and vegetables. Karen was able to change the negativities, both mentally and physically, by changing her diet. She states, "I feel very positive about life now! My husband and I are closer now, and my relationship with my children is stronger. I feel more at peace than I ever have before."

FERMENTATION

Did you know that education is necessary for proper digestion? It is imperative that a person learn which foods are "digestion compatible." Different foods require different time schedules. Mixing "incompatible foods" will result in some of them digesting while others lie and rot in the digestive tract, because they require a longer digestive period and different enzymes. The result is gas, stomachache, and many times, a feeling of lethargy. Health author Glen R. Shaw states in his book "Earning Good Health and Long Life": "Low energy and the need for extra sleep are sure signs that you need to change the food combinations you are eating." Mr. Shaw recounts an experience he had. "I can remember not long after I married, eating a lot of tuna fish sandwiches, and I soon went to the doctor, complaining of gas. He gave me some charcoal pills and said I was swallowing too much air as I ate. The trouble, of course, was eating meat and bread together, along with salad dressing. The bread stopped digesting when the stomach changed the pH to digest the tuna fish. The improperly digesting bread then started forming gas."

Digestion is the first step to converting food to energy. The digestive tract provides our bodies with the essential nutrients for survival. Digestion does not all take place in the stomach. The mouth, stomach, and small intestine all help digest food. Also, in the colon there will be some residue of nourishment to be absorbed. If we had the ability to see inside our stomachs, we might be more careful what we carelessly dump into it. Good health depends upon our body's ability to properly digest and assimilate food, distribute nutrients from the food and adequately eliminate waste from the bowels.

Health author Lee Du Belle, in her book "Proper Food Combining Cookbook" explains that:

- Acid fruit inhibits the flow of protein digestives

- Different proteins, eaten at the same time, confuse the timing of when to send the strongest and weakest digestive juices

- Fat inhibits the flow of protein digestives

- Sweet fruits inhibit the flow of protein digestives

THE CANDIDA CONNECTION

When fermentation occurs, sugars turn the undigested foods into an alcohol type of composition. This promotes the unchecked growth of the yeast organism, Candida Albicans. The excessive alcohol content which results from fermentation and Candida can actually make a person drunk! This sounds far-fetched, but it is true.

Dr. John H. Jeffries, M.D. states in the June 1986 issue of "Total Health": "Production of large amounts of alcohol causes one to become a living 'still' ... Production of large amounts of alcohol within the body causes even the non-drinker to become drunk ... an overgrowth of Candida albicans in the gastrointestinal tract ... produces systemic biochemical changes and, for want of a better term, 'blows' the immune system. It also sends out 'phony' signals to the glands, which cause the endocrine system to act as a free agent, without checks and balances. Alcohol is produced mainly by the fermentation of sugars and starches."

Other causes of fermentation: Other contributors to the fermentation process are (1) drinking fluids with meals, because the hydrochloric acid [Hcl] is diluted and cannot adequately breakdown the foods, and (2) eating just before you go to bed. The digestion slows way down or stops altogether. (3) Worry or negative emotions restrict proper digestion. DO NOT EAT WHILE YOU ARE UPSET. The food you eat will turn to poisons in your system.

DIGESTION DESTROYERS

AGING: Our stomach produces less HCL as we grow older. We have also destroyed the enzymes that produce HCL by the foods we eat. We can also have poor digestion and not be old.

ALCOHOL: Alcohol produces acid with a burning effect on the stomach lining, and causes inflammation. This is why alcoholics have gastritis problems.

ANTACIDS: They reduce HCL in the stomach and prevent protein from being digested. They will neutralize acids that are causing fermentation, but they also reduce the natural HCL production. More natural HCL is needed to treat the cause rather than the symptoms.

ANTIBIOTICS: They destroy the friendly bacterial flora in the colon. This causes deficiencies of the B-complex vitamins and vitamin K, and can lead to dysentery.

CHLORINATED WATER: Interferes with digestion. If digestion is a problem, change to pure water and the digestive formulas will work better.

COFFEE: Increases acid production, especially black without cream as a buffer.

COLA DRINKS: Contain phosphoric acid which signals the stomach that acid is already present, and it does not have to produce its own hydrochloric acid.

DIARRHEA: Interferes with proper digestion and causes nutritional problems.

LIQUIDS: Drinking liquids with meals. It dilutes HCL in the stomach so there isn't enough to digest food adequately.

MINERAL OIL: Keeps B-complex vitamins from being absorbed in the body. It destroys vitamin A.

NITROSAMINES: Form in the stomach by two food constituents, amines and nitrites. Cancer of the bladder, esophagus and stomach increase when they are present. Nitrites are more likely to be formed with the lack of hydrochloric acid.

PROCESSED FOOD: It is thought that one cause of gastric ulcers is processed food, lacking natural fiber and protein, but high in calories. Natural food is one of your best protections against stomach problems.

STRESS OR WORRY: These have an effect of reducing enzyme production. Don't eat when you are worried or under stress. If you need to eat, only eat food that is easy to digest.

FOOD COMBINATIONS: Wrong combinations of food can create indigestion and acid stomach. Proper food combining means eating foods that will digest well together. Protein and starch are a poor combination. Sugars should not be consumed with proteins or starch. Fruits should be eaten alone.

MORE FOOD FOR THOUGHT

Dr. William Donald Kelley, who was given The Humanitarian Award in 1975 by The International Association of Cancer Victims and Friends says, "No one in this society should eat protein without taking pancreatic enzymes at the same time. Pancreatic enzymes are the safest and cheapest insurance available against cancer."

He continues, "We find hydrochloric acid deficiencies very wide-spread, even among teenagers, so most people need this supplement, not just cancer patients. Moreover, among vegetarians hydrochloric acid deficiency is virtually universal. I've only found one vegetarian in all my years of practice who did not need this supplement."

Without proper digestion of food, assimilation and elimination of nutrients can seriously interfere with the proper function of the whole body. Minerals cannot be assimilated without sufficient HCL in our stomach. Dr. Kelley says, "To make sure your body absorbs the minerals properly, take hydrochloric acid tablets. Since mineral absorption is so important for a healthy pancreas, you could also consider hydrochloric acid tablets to be a cheap form of anti-cancer insurance—just like pancreatic enzyme tablets."

Food and stress are the root of digestive problems. The following ingredients are necessary in a good formula to increase the levels of HCL and improve protein assimilation, both vegetable and animal protein. There is probably no other combination of natural ingredients that can benefit the body more. The gastro-intestinal system needs support and these are nutrients that help the body utilize the food for a healthy body and mind. A large part of our population cannot produce the proper amount of pancreatic digestive enzymes and adding this important supplement to the diet improves digestion and health.

HYDROCHLORIC ACID: HCL is necessary for the assimilation of vitamins and minerals, especially vitamin C and calcium. It keeps bacteria under control. If the bacteria is not destroyed in the stomach it will interfere with the absorption of food nutrients. One of the primary causes of an overacid stomach is the lack of HCL. When missing or in low supply it allows the food to ferment, thus causing acids of fermentation which are many times more damaging to the stomach. This fermentation of acids can cause ulcers and gallbladder attacks.

HCL has been proven very effective in killing harmful bacteria. When traveling and eating different and stra⁻ ge food and water it should be a part of the daily diet. It has the ability to break down toxic elements. A professor A.E.

Austin claims HCL to have strong germicidal property and says the following, "When hydrochloric acid content of the gastric fluid is deficient or absent, grave results must gradually and inevitably appear in human metabolism. First of all, we shall have an increasing and gradual starvation of the mineral elements in the food supply. The food will be incompletely digested and failure of assimilation must occur.

"Secondly, a septic (pus forming toxins in the blood or tissues) process of the tissues will appear: pyorrhea, dyspepsia, nephritis, appendicitis, boils, abscesses, pneumonia, etc., will become increasingly manifested. Again, a normal gastric fluid demands activity of the gallbladder contents and of the pancreas for neutralization. Deficiency of normal acid leads to stagnation of these organs, causing diabetes and gallstones. In other words, an absence or a great deficiency of HCL gives rise to multitudinous degenerative reactions and prepares the way to all forms of degenerative disease."

PEPSIN is a natural enzyme that breaks down proteins and is dependent on the HCL contents. It is secreted by the stomach when HCL is present. Pepsin breaks down protein into smaller components so it can be absorbed.

PANCREATIN works as a catalyst to other protein digesting enzymes. It improves protein assimilation. It helps digestion throughout the gastrointestinal tract. It digests protein, starch and fats.

MYCOZYME: This enzyme also works as a catalyst and works with kipase and mylase in digestion of fat and complex carbohydrates. PAPAIN is a powerful protein digesting enzyme. It is from the papaya fruit. Its purpose is to break down the protein into amino acids. Papain contains proteolytic ferments which has the advantage of working in both acid and alkaline environments.

BROMELAIN is a natural vegetable enzyme. It is from pineapple. It has the ability to digest protein for better absorption.

BILE SALTS are essential for fat digestion. It stimulates the bile flow to combat constipation and improve gall bladder function. It is essential for fat absorption, including absorption of essential fatty acids and fat-soluble vitamins.

LIPASE is a natural aid in digestion of fat and complex carbohydrates.

You have heard the saying, "We are not what we eat, but what we assimilate." If we do not break foods down properly, they cannot be absorbed. Enzymes help digest foods.

Nutrients For Digestion

Antacids are big selling over-the-counter medications. Some doctors suggest taking them as calcium supplements. However, antacids may contain the following besides calcium: sodium, aluminum, mineral oil, talc, sugar, corn starch, corn syrup and food coloring.

It's cheaper to buy a calcium supplement, which may have other natural minerals along with it, than to use antacids as a source of this important mineral. Research has linked heavy aluminum-containing antacid use with symptoms of osteoporosis and may be responsible for other types of bone disorders. The safer and healthier route would be to take nutrients which will enhance digestion naturally.

Vitamin A—Promotes digestion and assimilation of food. Assists in maintaining normal glandular activity. Lack of Vitamin A can cause digestive and intestinal disturbances and decreased gastric acid.

Acidophilus—Increases the friendly bacteria in the colon, which are essential for the production of B vitamins. It helps to strengthen the immune system. It reduces toxic wastes in the large intestines.

Aloe Vera—Stimulates peristalsis only on the lower third of the colon. This is very important to keep it clean and free from worms and parasites. It is very useful for the irritated colon, as found in colitis and Crohn's disease. It is helpful in cases of heartburn as well as other gastrointestinal disorders.

Lemon Juice—Lemon juice is metabolized in the body to an alkaline ash. Lemons assist in cleansing the stomach and liver. Lemons are rich in potassium, vitamin C, bioflavonoids and calcium.

B-complex Vitamins—Niacin especially stimulates the function of hydrochloric acid and the amino acid lysine. All the B-complex vitamins are involved one way or another in promoting a healthy digestive tract. They help with appetite stimulation, digestion, assimilation and elimination. They assist enzymes in metabolism of proteins, fats and carbohydrates. The B vitamins help sustain normal function of the gastrointestinal tract.

Vitamin C—Detoxifies nitrates and also destroys nitrosamines that have already been formed.

Calcium—A very important mineral. Decreased absorption of it is linked to low hydrochloric acid in the stomach. This deficiency could lead to learning problems, hyperactivity and muscle spasms.

Catnip—This herb is called "nature's Alka-Seltzer." The Indians used it for infant colic. It has a sedative effect on the nervous system.

Comfrey and Pepsin—This combination is very effective in dissolving the mucus coating in the small intestine, where absorption of nutrients takes place. This coating is formed to protect itself from junk food, homogenized milk, pollutants and additives. The coating in the colon can become tough and thick as plastic. The pepsin is a digestive enzyme which works on the mucus, and the comfrey helps hold the pepsin to the intestinal wall so it can dissolve the mucus. This formula is also a digestive aid. The allantoin content helps produce healthy new cells, and is very nourishing.

Exercise—Very effective in helping the body produce lactic acid, which improves digestion.

Fiber—Fiber foods assist the function and absorption ability of the intestinal tract. Whole natural foods, water and exercise are very vital in maintaining the health of the digestive system.

Garlic—Neutralizes putrefactive toxins and kills bad bacteria. Eliminates gas and helps in digestion.

Gentian—Stimulates circulation and strengthens the system. It is usually used in digestive combinations for weakened muscular tone of the digestive organs.

Ginger—An excellent herb for indigestion as well as for stomach cramps. It is very effective as a cleansing agent through the bowels and kidneys. It is good for circulation and promotes perspiration.

Golden Seal—Contains antiseptic properties and acts as a tonic on the mucous membrane lining of the stomach. Always use in small amounts—it's more effective. It is useful for digestive problems such as gastritis, peptic ulcers and colitis. If a person has low blood sugar it is wise to substitute myrrh instead of golden seal.

Kefir and Yogurt—Aid digestion. The lactic acid acts as a cleanser as well as an antiseptic for the gastrointestinal tract. All types of pathogenic bacteria and harmful germs are killed within five hours of eating these foods.

Magnesium—Relaxes the gall bladder to help in pain and spasms. Aids in prevention of indigestion. Alkalizes the system. Reduces waste matter and aids in its elimination. Calms nerves. Activates enzymes.

Marshmallow—This relaxing herb will help reduce inflammation throughout the gastrointestinal tract.

Peppermint Oil—Excellent remedy for flatulence (gas). Add 8 drops of oil of peppermint to one pint of water. A drop or two can be placed on the tongue for good results.

Psyllium Powder—It cleans the colon. When taken with a liquid it creates bulk and pulls toxins from the intestines and colon. It cleans the gastrointestinal tract to provide better digestion.

Water—Pure water helps keep the gall bladder healthy. Too little water can cause gallstones to develop, which are usually a combination of fats and calcium.

Zinc—Stimulates the digestive cells to release the contents necessary for the conversion of digestive enzymes from the inactive form to the active.

The Role of Enzymes, Amino Acids

ENZYMES

The word enzyme is derived from the word "enzymos" which means "fermented" or "leaven" (to make a change) in Greek.

Enzymes are protein-like substances, formed in plants and animals. They act as catalysts in chemical reactions. Enzymes are vital to health. They help speed up processes in the body which normally would take place very slowly or not at all.

Glands and organs depend upon enzymatic activity and cannot function properly without enzymes. Enzymes exist in all living things. There are 700 different enzymes at work in the body. Each one performs a different job. If the body is missing even one enzyme, there is a risk of failing health. When we obtain enough enzymes from the food we eat, they help provide boundless energy. However, enzymes can only be obtained from raw, live foods. This makes the body work hard to try and manufacture the missing enzymes and overworks the glands. This can throw the glands out-of-balance and causes a person to feel fatigued and exhausted. This is why people who consume large quantities of cooked proteins and starches, and very little enzyme-rich fruits and vegetables, are often tired and have little "pep".

There are four main categories of food enzymes:

1. Lipase (which serves to break down fat)

2. Protease (which breaks down protein)

3. Cellulase (which assists in breaking down cellulose)

4. Amylase (which breaks down starch)

If we do not get sufficient enzymes, we will age faster. This is because our bodies' enzyme production slows down. Therefore, enzymes can be called "the keys to the fountain of youth".

ENZYME-KILLERS

1. Fluoridated water paralyzes enzymes.

2. Food cooked above 118 degrees kills live enzymes.

3. Exposure to air and light dissipates enzymes. If you ever see a pale, limp vegetable do not eat it! Of course, you probably wouldn't, anyway ... but the above describes an enzyme-depleted food.

4. Long-term storage at room temperature or above diminishes enzymatic activity. The food is half-dead by the time you eat it; and enzymes are only present in live food. Refrigerated food keeps a little longer, but it is best to eat it as fresh as possible. Sprouted beans, grains and seeds provide a treasure-trove of enzymes. Be sure to include plenty of fresh fruits, vegetables, their juices, and sprouted foods for health and vitality!

AMINO ACIDS

Amino acids are the building blocks of proteins. Proteins are substances which occur in all living matter. A proper balance of amino acids can benefit the blood, the skin, the immune system and digestive system. Amino acids also can help with neurotransmitters in the brain, helping to stabilize moods and balance the thinking process.

Health expert Carlson Wade observes, "A missing amino acid is like a missing building block. The entire structure may threaten to collapse because of a single weakness. For example, you may enjoy a corn-based diet, but corn is deficient in tryptophan, and this deficiency can cause emotional disorders and insomnia. If you add grains, seeds or nuts to corn, you will provide the tryptophan necessary for brain nourishment."

There are eight essential amino acids and twenty-four complementary ones, which work synergistically to promote health throughout the entire body. Carnitine is an example of an amino acid which helps metabolize fat and reduce triglycerides. Carnitine is synthesized from the combination of the amino acids lysine and methionine.

Methionine helps remove heavy metals from the tissues. Lead is one heavy metal which causes brain damage. We are exposed to it through industrial and metropolitan pollution. Measures have been taken in recent years to reduce the amount of lead from various sources, but it is still a problem; it emits from factory smokestacks, cars, etc. It is present in any industrialized setting. A folk remedy for accumulated lead in the body is the ingestion of baked beans. Beans contain sulfur-bearing amino acids, which have a chelating effect upon toxic substances including lead.

THE PROTEIN MYTH

For many years—until recently, in fact—it was believed that you had to eat a complete protein at one meal in order for the body to utilize it properly.

However, it has been discovered that if you eat complementary proteins throughout the day, the body will assimilate it and extract the amino acids it needs to regenerate its daily protein requirements for blood, enzyme, hormone and antibody production. Most of the twenty-two amino acids needed for protein synthesis can be manufactured by the body. Eight cannot. These eight "essential amino acids" must be supplied through diet. The body can only utilize a measured portion of protein at any one time. Excess amino acids, whether they are from incomplete or complete proteins, are excreted in the urine. Therefore, a major portion of that big steak dinner is just a waste of money; it basically serves to gratify the taste buds.

There are many other myths which have been propagated throughout this century, primarily by vested interests in the food industry. Meat and dairy councils have financed advertising which heavily emphasizes animal products as major components of a healthy diet. However, today commercial beef and chicken contain concentrated amounts of synthetic hormones, pesticides, antibiotics, etc., and these have harmful effects on the people who eat them.

Proteins from plant sources are more easily assimilated than the protein found in meats, which the body must arduously process in order to obtain any protein benefits. Thus, a person can experience more sustained energy while digesting fruits, vegetables, seeds and herbs than while attempting to metabolize animal tissues.

The concentrated synthetic hormones found in animal products such as milk, cheese and eggs can influence precocious puberty changes in children. Excessive estrogen from these sources, when not eliminated by the liver, can lead to breast cancer, as well as cancer of the reproductive system and many other problems. A diet rich in B-complex vitamins, especially choline and inositol, will help the liver to process the excessive estrogen into "estriol", an anticarcinogen.

Protein requirements for the body can be met if you obtain a sufficient amount of calories from a wide variety of vegetables, grains, legumes and fruits. Too much protein from a high-animal source diet can leave toxic residues of metabolic wastes in the tissues, constipation, autotoxemia, hyperacidity, nutritional deficiencies, accumulations of uric acid, intestinal putrefaction, arthritis, gout, kidney damage, schizophrenia, atherosclerosis, heart disease and cancer; even premature aging and a shorter life expectancy. Excessive protein in the diet can also cause a negative calcium balance which can pave the way for demineralization of bones or osteoporosis.

Complete proteins in a given day can be supplied by these combinations: corn and beans; rice and beans; grains and legumes; grains and seeds; or seeds and legumes. Of course, varying amounts of amino acids are found in most natural foods. Avoiding junk foods and concentrating on a nutritious diet will ensure that your body utilizes the protein efficiently.

Some people experience a "craving" for meat and interpret this feeling as their body's need for this type of food. People who stop eating red meat may experience withdrawal symptoms at first, and then as their bodies get rid of the poisons contained in it, the craving disappears. (Did you know that eating 12 ounces of char-broiled steak in one week is equivalent to smoking two packs of cigarettes a day for that same period?) If you cannot stop eating meat completely, then try eating it sparingly, as a complement to your meals rather than the dominating food. The Orientals are, as a group, very healthy. Maybe it is because their diets include plentiful amounts of grains and vegetables, with little meat. Besides the fact that a high meat diet is detrimental to health, it is also more expensive on the grocery bill. For additional delicious meatless recipes, please read my book "Today's Healthy Eating".

ACID/ALKALINE

Even though it is recommended that protein and starch foods are not included in the same meal, nature combines these two substances proportionately in grains, seeds and vegetables in a manner which is digestible. When man eats proteins and starches in the same meal, they are in a concentrated form and do not assimilate well together. This is because proteins require an acid medium for digestion, and carbohydrates (starches and sugars) need an alkaline medium for this purpose. An improper combination upsets the digestive system and causes gas and bloating and a lethargic feeling.

According to health expert Dr. William Howard Hay, acid to alkaline foods should be balanced 1 to 4. Alkaline foods include all vegetables and fruits (except plums and cranberries); also almonds and sprouts made from seeds, grains and beans.

Acid foods include animal proteins (meat, fish, shellfish, eggs, cheese, poultry, nuts (except almonds); also foods made from cereal starches and sugars).

CHOLESTEROL ...
the liver, bowels, gall bladder's role in regulating cholesterol

Your body needs cholesterol. It manufactures it from the natural oils and fats we ingest. The body is able to synthesize cholesterol for important purposes, yet keep it under control so that it does not become excessive, by manufacturing lecithin. Lecithin is the "cholesterol regulator" which the body will make from nutrients in the diet. In nature, lecithin and cholesterol always accompany each other. An egg contains both of these substances, therefore keeping each other in balance.

Cholesterol serves many important functions ... it helps build cell walls; assists in the synthesis of pituitary and sex hormones; it is used by the adrenal glands, the brain and the myelin sheaths which protect the nerves—(almost 25% of all the cholesterol in the human body is contained in the brain and spinal cord); it is made into bile acids to help metabolize fats and fat-soluble vitamins; vitamin D can be synthesized in the body from cholesterol and assists in the metabolism of calcium.

CHOLESTEROL "SCARE"

The big cholesterol "scare" is a distortion of information. *There is no correlation between eating cholesterol-rich foods and blood cholesterol levels.* These levels are entirely dependent upon the body's ability to take care of it through the liver, gall bladder and bowels. Health author Sue Moody states in her book "Cholesterol Confusion ... Who is Responsible": "How did our ancestors and their ancestors survive and thrive on a diet filled with such foods as lard, eggs, butter and red meats? If the fat in the diet is the reason for high cholesterol and the cause of heart disease, then our civilization would not be in existence today, because before the third decade of this century the daily diet consisted almost entirely of animal fats, and cholesterol-rich foods ... Heredity may be a major factor of high cholesterol and if this be the case, the amount of dietary cholesterol ingested would have no correlation whatsoever on lowering the cholesterol levels in the blood."

Eight foods that have been shown to lower cholesterol are eggplant, garlic, fiber, apples, beans, yogurt, oat bran, and psyllium. Other foods and supplements which do this also are: salmon oil, evening primrose oil, olive oil, kelp, scullcap, goldenseal, hawthorn berries, barley, carrots, cayenne pepper, onions and lecithin.

Another health writer, David Skousen, writes: "Cholesterol is harmful if, instead of lubricating the walls of the body's blood vessels, it begins to stick to them and build up fatty deposits that also injure the sides of the vessel walls."

"To keep cholesterol in a safe condition, the body is able to create a substance that emulsifies cholesterol. In other words, it is broken up and disbursed so that it won't coagulate and adhere to the artery walls. This naturally-occurring substance is called phospholipids, and is a mixture of phosphorus and lipid fats. Another name is lecithin."

Excessive sugar intake can produce high triglyceride levels even in a healthy individual. Mr. Skousen explains it this way: "The most abundant lipid of animal tissues is the triglyceride, but when people consume too many simple carbohydrates (sugar), they flood into the blood, requiring the liver to convert them into a triglyceride type of fat. These fats are called triglycerides because the liver hooks three fatty acids (tri) to a sugar or glycerine molecule (glyceride).

However, too many of these thicken the blood and they can pile up and block capillaries or even arteries leading to vital tissues."

"There are two or three different forms of triglycerides, depending on who does the dividing. The body packages them with cholesterol and protein so they can ride the bloodstream better—since water and oil don't mix."

"These packages are named 'lipoproteins.' The biggest package has the very lowest density (VLDL). The middle package has a low density (LDL). But the smallest has the highest density of all (HDL), a very strange arrangement of opposites."

"VLDL packages carry most of the triglycerides in the blood and seem to be the most dangerous to artery health. LDL and HDL packages carry most of the cholesterol. It was finally discovered that those with the highest blood HDL's had the fewest heart attacks. Surprisingly, this had been known by scientists for over 35 years, but hardly anybody gave it any attention! This was because cholesterol phobia branded its carrier as the bad boy. It was a case of guilt by association. Yet currently, HDL's are 'in.'"

Excessive cholesterol can be eliminated via the bile (which is made by the liver). It is then discharged through the gall bladder into the bowels. Next it may be reabsorbed into the blood or the body will excrete it. (The reabsorbed cholesterol can be metabolized by the cells and reduced to carbon dioxide and water.)

So, you see, the body has its own method for balancing cholesterol levels, as long as it is kept well-nourished, and the organs are functioning properly.

Digestive Disorders

When a person's digestion goes awry, all sorts of problems can result. Allergies are connected with digestive disorders and both are interrelated with many ailments.

ALLERGIES

Many people cannot enjoy eating certain foods because they are allergic to them. What causes sensitivities to foods? Some experts believe that when a specific type of food is the main component of a diet, that the body develops a peculiar reaction to it and rebels. The substances to which the body is sensitive are called "allergens" because they provoke the allergic response. It is believed that these allergens irritate the system because they are made up of protein molecules which are bigger than those found normally in foods. When the blood vessels and mucous membranes are healthy they "screen out" the larger protein molecules. They are able to do this because of their finely knit structures. However, the blood vessel and membrane tissues of the allergic person are poor quality and allow the entry of the larger protein molecules. When the tissues of the body are irritated by these allergens, or molecules, the body releases a chemical known as "histamine". This substance causes the mucous membranes to swell, and if the irritation is extensive the entire body can be affected, with subsequent swellings of the arms, legs, etc.

Allergies have been linked to the usual red eyes, sniffles, but also to mental illness, fatigue, insomnia and a host of gastrointestinal disorders.

Allergic reactions are associated with lowered immune system function. Normally, the "T" cells of the immune system takes care of unwanted "invaders." When the immune system is not operating efficiently, the "T" cells may be small in number or are unable to recognize invaders from normal substances and attack everything. When there is chaos in the immune system, allergies can be one of the results. Health expert Paavo Airola, Ph.D., has stated: "The solution for digestive problems caused by allergies is as simple as it is difficult to implement: all allergens must be eliminated from the diet for a certain period, which must often extend for years, to give the body time to "forget" about them. Fasting is an excellent way to begin the treatment. Prolonged juice fasting, or repeated short fasts, will eventually result in better tolerance of previous allergens. After juice fasting, the patient can try a mono diet—one food, which he knows he tolerates well, at a time. Then he can add one new food each week, testing it for a week. If the body's reaction is good, this food is kept in the diet and another new food is added—if the reaction is bad, that food should be discarded and a new food tried. This way all real allergens can be eliminated from the diet."

Stress can lower immunity and resistance to disease. It can also wreak havoc in the digestive system. There is a true story of an army surgeon from the 1700s, William Beaumont, who noticed a wound in a patient's stomach which did not heal after several weeks. His patient, Alexis St. Martin, was a sort of guinea pig, as the inquisitive surgeon used a glass rod to touch the inside of the man's stomach and observe the metabolic reactions to digestion and stress. Dr. Beaumont recorded that "the lining of the stomach had a soft, or velvet-like appearance ... With fear, anger, or whatever depresses the nervous system—the villous coat of the stomach becomes red and dry, at other times pale and moist."

Food addictions and binges are part of the food allergy syndrome. Health author Annemarie Colbin explains in her book *Food and Healing*: "We are addicted to a food or drink (and thus crave it) when (a) the food creates symptoms of imbalances, such as headache, fatigue, skin problems, digestive disorders, or tension, some time after ingestion, and (b) the symptoms can be relieved by consuming more of the same food. If, for example, you give up sweets or coffee, you will initially crave them and feel generally depressed and tense. Eat a cookie, have a cup of coffee, and the symptoms go away—although not the addiction."

"A food allergy is the opposite of addiction: Unpleasant symptoms appear almost immediately upon consumption of the offending substance and are best controlled by avoiding that substance completely. There are many instances, however, when we do not connect our allergic symptoms with our food intake. We'll continue to crave the allergen and suffer through fatigue, tension and headaches without realizing what their cause is or how simply they could be cured."

Cravings for foods are caused by imbalances in the body, which it is trying to correct. If we consume too many alkaline-forming foods, the body will manifest the imbalance by a craving for acid-forming foods. The cravings for the opposite, or complementary foods do not always show up for foods with high nutritional value. Sometimes the cravings are for sugary sweets, coffee, alcohol or other detrimental foods. (You have probably read about kids who will eat dirt because their bodies are lacking some of the trace minerals which are found in soil.) The key to good health and avoiding allergies is a varied diet, with plenty of nutrients. The Chinese call the balance in the body and in the foods we eat "Yin" and "Yang". They are taught from childhood which foods are yin and which foods are yang, and when there is an imbalance in the body they instinctively eat the foods which have the balancing effect.

There are gastrointestinal disorders associated with food allergies. They include: celiac disease, Crohn's disease, colitis, and colic.

Celiac disease—This disease has been connected to sensitivity to wheat gluten, soybeans, eggs and milk. Some experts feel that the gluten intolerance may be triggered by ingestion of cow's milk during infancy, which has permanently damaged the intestinal tract.

Crohn's disease—This is a severe illness, characterized by colon inflammation. It has also been linked to gluten intolerance. *Foods with even the tiniest bit of gluten must be eliminated from the diet.*

Colitis—Allergens which are known to provoke colitis include milk, eggs, chocolate, meat, nuts, wheat, corn and citrus foods. There are cases of chronic ulcerative colitis which have gone into remission when dairy products were eliminated from the diet.

Colic—Infant colic has been eradicated when cow's milk has been eliminated from the breast-feeding mother's diet.

Another disorder connected with the gastrointestinal tract which is important to mention is "hiatal hernia". In his book *Hiatal Hernia Syndrome: Insidious Link to Major Illness*, Dr. Theodore A. Baroody explains: "Large portions of the population experience this disorder at one time or another in their lives—I estimate as high as 85%. It is an insidious masquerader that paves the way to many other serious disorders. I call it the Hiatal Hernia Syndrome. *Hiatus* is the special hole in the diaphragm, the breathing muscle, through which the esophagus normally passes to become the stomach. *Hernia* is the term for a weakened—in this case, stretched—muscle. If, for any reason, the diaphragmatic muscle is weakened or torn, the stomach will be forced upward through the diaphragm, creating the problematical condition..." Hiatal hernias cause all types of digestive disorders, including: regurgitation, vomiting, bloating, diarrhea, constipation, intestinal gas, belching, hiccups, nausea, heartburn, and colic in children, plus many other symptoms.

The Healthy Way To Eat

Fruit in the morning ... Fresh fruits are the "cleansers" of the body. Their high water content helps wash many toxins and impurities out of the system.

The live enzymes in fruit facilitate digestion and promote energy in the body. However, if combined with other foods they are unable to pass through the system as they were designed to do. They cause fermentation, indigestion and gas. Cooked fruit promotes an acid condition in the body, and thus becomes an acid-forming food. (Do not confuse acid foods with acid-forming foods.) Some acid foods (such as fresh fruit) actually help neutralize acidity in the body, as they become alkaline-forming once they are inside.

It take more energy for the body to digest foods than to perform any other function. In the morning you need all the energy you can muster to start your day! Therefore, it makes sense that you eat a fruit meal, or drink fresh fruit juice ... for easy digestion and energy for morning demands. All fruit in season, and tree-ripened fruit contain all the nutrients the human body needs to sustain itself.

Do not clog your body with hard-to-digest proteins and carbohydrates. During the period of time during the night when your body is without food it goes through a cleanse. Sleep is also a detoxifier. This is also when healing takes place because the body's energies can be directed to that instead of to digestion. Our bodies go through a type of fast while we sleep. When we eat in the morning we break our fast, hence, the name "breakfast." Toxins accumulate in the stomach and your first food in the morning should be a cleansing food. As mentioned in this book, take half of a fresh lemon squeezed in a glass of water, one hour or more before breakfast. Some people, such as those with hypoglycemia, diabetes or candida, cannot handle large amounts of fructose. Those with serious candida problems should avoid all fruit until further healing takes place. Some people who have had severe reactions to fruit find that it is the spray on the fruit, rather than the fruit itself, that cause the problem. People who cannot handle large quantities of fruit should start out slowly with fruit in the morning. It is suggested that they eat half of a fruit such as a banana or apple, and see how it is tolerated. Persons with the above conditions should avoid fruits with high sugar content, such as grapes and dried fruit—raisins and dates.

Nutritionists Harvey and Marilyn Diamond remind us in their book *Fit for Life*: "The human body is not designed to digest more than one concentrated food in the stomach at the same time ... Any food that is not a fruit and is not a vegetable is concentrated."

Why do you get sleepy after a protein and carbohydrate meal? Try eating a fruit meal and then taking a nap. Do you see the difference? You can reach your own conclusion which one helps you to stay awake!

Vegetables and protein for lunch ... We do not advocate staying away from meat completely. However, meat should be a complementary, not a dominating food, in combination with vegetables. In other words, vegetables should constitute the major portion of the meal. They should be raw or lightly steamed. A vegetable salad with chicken or tuna is delicious! Or try your hand at Oriental cooking. The Chinese have realized for years the benefits of this type of eating. Most Chinese are healthy and thin.

There are many variations to the vegetable/protein approach. You need not become bored. For mouth-watering sample dishes, turn to the recipe section in this book.

Vegetables and grains for dinner ... Vegetables and grains are very compatible. Vegetables contain all of the body-building minerals needed by the body. It can synthesize some vitamins, but we must obtain minerals from our foods.

Grains contain amino acids, minerals and supply roughage or fiber. This is very important for the health of the colon and entire digestive system.

Some people are sensitive to the gluten in wheat. Health expert Dr. Bernard Jensen, D.C., Ph.D., suggests that rice (which is gluten-free), rye (which builds muscle), and cornmeal (also gluten-free), are excellent grains. He says that "one of the finest wheat substitutes is millet. When I went to the Hunza Valley, I found these old men died at 120 with every tooth in their head ... they had plenty of calcium, and they were living on a lot of millet."

FOOD COMBINING

"Keep it simple, sweetheart." Do you remember that cliche? It usually refers to something else, but in this case it is wise to remember when eating. You will feel better and have more energy when you combine foods properly, yet eat simply. Actor Michael Landon shares his ideas: "Eat only what you really need and only when you are actually hungry. Keep your meals simple, with just a few items from two or three of the basic food groups. You feel good after a simple meal."

We have been taught that a balanced diet is one providing many different foods at one meal, but actually we are serving an imbalanced meal. Too many different foods at one time can cause poor absorption, improper digestion, fermentation in the colon and cause heartburn and gas; also the formation of toxins.

Simple preparation of food will assure proper digestion, assimilation and elimination.

Proper food combining starts with a glass of water with a half of lemon first thing in the morning. This cleans the stomach and helps the liver to get into action. Fresh fruit, cereal, seeds, or nuts can be eaten later on for breakfast. Lunch can consist of a fresh vegetable salad, nuts, vegetables, and rice. A fresh salad, steamed vegetables and baked potatoes are delicious for supper.

It is best if no protein foods are eaten after 2 p.m. It is hard for the body to digest protein in the evening and it can cause fermentation.

The following are guidelines for healthy eating and proper food combining:

1. Eat acids and starches at separate meals.

2. Eat protein foods and carbohydrate foods at separate meals.

3. Eat but one concentrated protein food at a meal.

4. Eat proteins and acids at separate meals.

5. Eat fats and proteins at separate meals.

6. Eat sugars and proteins at separate meals.

7. Eat starches and sugars at separate meals.

Even though it is recommended that protein and starch foods are not blended in the same meal, nature skillfully combines these two substances proportionately in grains, seeds, and vegetables in a manner which is digestible. When man eats proteins and starches in the same meal, they are in a concentrated form and do not assimilate well together. This is because proteins require an acid medium for digestion, and carbohydrates (starches and sugars) need an alkaline medium for this purpose. An improper combination upsets the digestive system and causes gas and bloating and a lethargic feeling.

High protein foods and grains are usually acid-forming foods. There must be a balance between acid-forming foods and alkaline-forming foods in the diet. According to health expert, Dr. William Howard Hay, acid to alkaline foods should be balanced one to four. Alkaline foods include all vegetables and fruits (except plums and cranberries); also almonds.

Acid foods include animal proteins (meat, fish, shellfish, eggs, cheese, poultry, nuts (except almonds); also food made from cereal starches and sugars).

Most nutritionists agree that it is wise to only take milk products by themselves.

The above may scare you into thinking, "What can I eat?" However, the following are easy charts to which you can refer.

EASY FOOD COMBINING

The following are foods which can be eaten together.

Green Vegetables		Fat		Protein		Protein (Fat)		Protein
(non-starch)		Butter		Beef		Avocado		(Starch)
Asparagus	*Eat with*	Cream	*or*	Chicken	*or*	Cheese	*or*	Beans, dry
Bell pepper		Margarine		Duck		Kefir		peas, dry
Beets (top)		Oil		Egg		Nuts		
Broccoli				Goose		(no chestnuts		
Brussels Sprouts		*and*		Lamb		or peanuts)		
Cabbage				Pork		olives		
Cauliflower		Starch		Rabbit		sour cream		
Celery		Bread		Seafood		whole milk		
Cucumber		Cereal		Turkey		yogurt		
Dandelion		Corn						
Eggplant		Crackers						
Endive		Pasta						
Garlic		Potatoes						
Green Beans		Pumpkin						
Kale		Rice						
Lettuce		Squash						
Mushrooms								
Onion		*and*						
Parsley								
Peas, Fresh		Mild Starch						
Radishes		Beets						
Spinach		Carrots						
Sprouts		Parsnips						
Squash (no Hubbard)		Rutabagas						
Swiss Chard		Turnips						
Zucchini								

This chart shows that you can eat the non-starch green vegetables with fats, starches and mild starches (combined). Or you may eat the non-starch green vegetables in conjunction with regular protein, or with protein/fat or with protein/starch, but not with all of these combined.

The Healthy Way To Eat

Fruit, Sweet/Dried
Apricot
Banana
Date
Fig
Peach
Pear
Pineapple
Prune
Raisins
(Eat separate)

Fruit, Sweet/Fresh
Banana
Black Currant
Mango
Papaya
Persimmon
Grape
(Eat separate)

Melon
Cantaloupe
Casaba
Crenshaw
Honeydew
Muskmelon
Watermelon
(Eat separate)

Syrup, Sugar
Brown Sugar
Honey
Malt
Maple Syrup
Molasses
White Sugar
(Eat separate)

Fruit (Acid)
Acerola Cherry
Apple, (sour)
Cranberry
Currants
Gooseberries
Grapefruit
Sour Grapes
Kumquats
Lemons
Limes
Loganberries
Oranges
Pineapple
Plum, (sour)
Pomegranate
Tangerine
Tomato
(Eat separate)

Fruit (Sub-acid)
Apple
Apricot
Blackberries
Blueberries
Boysenberries
Cherries (sweet)
Nectarine
Peach (sweet)
Pear
Plum
Raspberries
(Eat separate)

Milk
(Separate from everything else)

This chart shows that fruits in the different categories need to be eaten alone, for they require different digestive enzymes in order to be assimilated. Do not eat fruit with any other types of foods.

Milk is to be ingested separately from all foods.
Sugars are to be eaten alone.

DIGESTION TIME

The digestion time of various foods is determined by how easy they are to assimilate by the body. Foods which are easily digested are often referred to as "mild foods" since they do not require a lot of work and energy to digest. The following are approximate timetables for digestion:

Green Vegetables (non-starch)—5 hours
Raw Juices—15 minutes
Fat—12 hours
Protein (meat)—12 hours
Protein (fat)—12 hours
Protein (starch)—12 hours
Starch—5 hours
Mild Starch—5 hours
Fruit, Sweet/Dried—3 hours
Fruit (Acid)—2 hours
Fruit (Sub-acid)—2 hours
Fruit, Sweet/Fresh—3 hours
Melon—2 hours
Syrup, Sugar—2 hours
Milk—12 hours

WEIGHT LOSS AND FOOD COMBINING

Have you said to yourself, "I can eat anything". "Thank goodness I was born with a strong stomach." Have you known someone that burps and belches and complains of a "bad stomach?" Did you ever think that that person once said he or she had a strong stomach and felt that they could eat anything and everything they wanted to without digestive problems?

In the meantime, you go on eating as you please without regards to your digestive system and one day your stomach rebels. Not only does your stomach rebel but you notice that you are gaining weight! You notice that when you eat meat and potatoes and top it off with a sweet dessert your stomach reacts violently. You also notice that you are constantly constipated. You wonder, "what is going on, I have always had a strong stomach, this cannot be happening to me."

Overloading the stomach and wrong food combining are the major causes of overweight, in my opinion. It is also the major cause of most diseases, along with constipation.

Many people are finding that their digestive troubles: their ailing gall bladders, malfunctioning livers, or disordered intestines, have been acquired because of improper food combining.

Nature cannot be fooled. If you eat large meals day in and day out and combine wrong foods, your stomach is bound to enlarge, and stretch to two or three times its normal size. There are natural laws we must obey in order to have good health and normal weight. The body cannot handle wrong chemical conditions that disrupt normal digestion. If you eat too much of a certain kind of food, the digestive system has to overwork and the tissues connected with it can become inflamed. This sometimes takes a long time, over a period of years, but it will show wear and tear on the organs and tissues.

It is possible to build up a tolerance to incompatible mixtures of food. This is what most of us have done who have not been trained in proper eating habits. This leads to depletion of energy and does damage to the tissues and organs of the body. This weakens our whole system and causes us mental and physical diseases, which are very common.

Weight loss is the reward we achieve when we properly combine our food, and eat less. We have more energy, and as we gain this energy it gives us the desire to eat properly. This type of weight loss is gradual and permanent.

Herbs Versus Drugs

Modern medicinal treatments are losing their credibility. There are too many adverse reactions from pharmaceutical drugs. These drugs are focused on the disease after it invades the body. These create havoc with the immune system. Antibiotics are fast coming to a close. There are so many of them, and now viruses and bacteria have built resistance to almost all antibiotics.

The widespread use of vaccinations and antibiotics is considered one of the main causes of immune system disorders. Dr. Robert Mendelsohn said, "there is a growing suspicion that immunization against relatively harmless childhood diseases may be responsible for the dramatic increase in autoimmune diseases since mass inoculations were introduced."

Autoimmune diseases are the epidemic plagues of our times. A large part of the population of the United States suffers from one or more of these disorders chronically. As long as we play games with the immune system and interfere with the body's only protection, we will see more and more unusual autoimmune diseases than we ever would have dreamed possible.

With all of these new diseases, the orthodox doctors, using drugs, are trying to put a monopoly on its methods of treatment. It is unconstitutional. Benjamin Rush, M.D., a signer of the Declaration of Independence, said: "The Constitution of this Republic should make special provisions for medical freedom, as well as religious freedom. To restrict the art of healing to one class of men and deny equal privileges to others will constitute the Bastille of medical science. All such laws are un-American and despotic."

A pamphlet put out by the government is entitled: "Assessing the Efficacy and Safety of Medical Technologies." It says, "it has been estimated that only 10-20 percent of all procedures currently used in medical practice have been shown to be efficacious by controlled trial." (This pamphlet can be obtained from the U.S. Office of Technology Assessment for Publication #PB286-929.)

Organized medicine is virtually a monopoly. Its members are quick to silence, discredit and destroy people or organizations who offer approaches that do not ring up profits for its interests. The concern is that organized medicine ultimately seeks to outlaw our freedom of choice. They are trying to take our constitutional rights away from us. (Proving Orthodox Medicine is Unproven by Coalition for Alternatives in Nutrition and Healthcare, Inc.)

Organized medicine attacks any alternate health care by accusing it of quackery. What is quackery? According to their own definition, if orthodox medicine is 80 percent unproven then they themselves are quacks! I believe the American Medical Association should be more humble in their approach to what is either valid or "quackery" in the field of nutrition. It is a well-known fact that the medical doctors lack nutritional education. Why should the A.M.A. be permitted to manipulate the government to prosecute alternative health care professionals who are helping people find better health and happiness?

Most of us in the health field are not against medical doctors. In fact, we are grateful for them and have used them many times. We just want our freedom to choose the type of health care we want. According to statistics gathered during the doctors' strikes in 1973, 1976, and 1978, it was proven that their absence decreased death rates.

In Israel in 1973 there was a 29-day physicians' strike and 50% fewer deaths were reported by the Jerusalem Burial Society. In 1976 a 52-day strike showed a 35% decrease in deaths in Bogota, Columbia, confirmed by the Morticians Association of Columbia. In 1978 Great Britain reported fewer deaths when doctors went on strike.

Yes! I feel doctors should be more humble when criticizing people for wanting to help themselves.

Modern drugs are powerful and quick to help remove the symptoms of disease. This action gives temporary relief, sometimes. Maybe there are times when we need this quick action. At least we need to have a free choice in deciding what action we will take. Drugs lead to more serious diseases later, as well as cause serious side effects. They are foreign substances to the human body. When a child is vaccinated, the body usually tries to eliminate it quickly by creating a fever, which is how the body eliminates foreign material. Drugs will not assimilate into the body's health-building metabolism. The body finds it hard to get rid of them once they are there. They accumulate in various organs and tissues to continue their negative side-effects.

I have heard the medical profession say if someone uses herbs they are self-diagnosing and the public is not capable of self-diagnosis. They say we are not capable of knowing what our bodies need. Some doctors have called herbs primitive and backwards and call drugs advanced and modern. There are birth defects caused by using drugs. This is advancement in medical technology? Have you ever heard of birth defects from using herbs?

Some doctors say that herbal treatments are really an uncontrolled form of drug therapy, that they are drugs because the average herb contains five or six drugs. Scientists have confirmed that whole herbs in their natural state are compatible to the body system and are accepted as food. We know that many drugs are derived from herbs. The problem arises when they remove part of an herb and do not use the part that prevents side-effects. The whole herb is designed to work together. I want to mention at this time that herbalists use only the herbs that are good for the body. Herbs are easily utilized to strengthen and

balance, and nourish the body system and are completely eliminated, leaving
behind health-building properties. The body has the knowledge to take from the
herbs what it needs and disregard the rest, without side effects. The body does
not know drugs, that is why there are so many side effects.

DRUGS AND THEIR SIDE EFFECTS

Dr. Paul Lofholm, Consultant to the National Institute for Drug Abuse said
the following: "... Everyone knows that children need different dosages of drugs
than adults. But it's only now being recognized that the adult dosages of most
drugs should usually be cut in half for an older person because they absorb and
excrete the drug at a much slower rate." Specialists often treat various diseases
not knowing what other doctors have prescribed. The medications can have
adverse reactions when combined. It has been estimated that a million
Americans diagnosed as senile really suffer from a misuse of prescribed drugs,
including large and harmful drug combinations. The dosages are much too high,
and combinations of drugs from different doctors, together can produce
symptoms diagnosed as senility. (From the National Institute For Drug Abuse.)

HOW SAFE ARE DRUGS

Prozac is another widely prescribed drug for depression. Side effects from
taking this anti-depressant range from: skin rash, itching, headache,
nervousness, insomnia, drowsiness, tremors, dizziness, fatigue, impaired
concentration, altered taste, nausea, vomiting, diarrhea and sexual impairment
to fever, weakness, joint pain and swelling, swollen lymph glands, and fluid
retention. A more serious consequence of taking this drug has recently been
publicized. It has been linked to suicide attempts and murders. It is believed to
induce violent and persistent suicidal and homicidal tendencies in many people
who otherwise would not even contemplate such behavior.

A so-called quick solution to restlessness and "hyperactivity" in children is, in
many instances, prescribed in the form of a drug called Ritalin. Ritalin has been
dubbed the `behavior pill'. Its slang names include Qualudes, Soupers and 714
ludes. Possible side effects may be: stunted growth, seizures in children prone to
them, sometimes blurring of vision, also nervousness, insomnia, skin rashes and
nausea.

One woman said her son's teacher badgered her until she agreed to take her
son to a doctor. The physician put the boy on Ritalin in the daytime and an anti-
depressant by night. The behavior of this ten-year-old boy did not change. Also,
his grades plummeted and he developed suicidal tendencies.

Remember when "interferon" was shouted as a miracle drug for cancer? Drug
companies began producing interferon artificially. It is one of the body's own
natural immune system chemicals which it produces by itself. It enhances the

body's own defensive and healing mechanism. It is a stress and disease resistance factor. It seems to diminish when you take aspirin and probably other drugs. It was said to be especially effective as a protective factor against cancer. Interferon is another chemical drug that backfired. Ironically, after all the shouting, artificial interferon has proven very disappointing, showing anti-cancer action in only 10 to 20 percent of cancer patients, and most of that was temporary. What can naturally be produced in the body cannot be produced synthetically. A study released in April 19, 1982 showed that artificial interferon may increase the ability of cancer cells to spread into normal tissues.

Vitamin C helps to produce natural interferon in the body. Many herbs contain large amounts of vitamin C.

One recent study showed that Licorice Root actually stimulates the interferon production in the body. Kelp, Burdock, Capsicum, Pau D'Arco, Red Clover, Chaparral and many herbs help to protect the immune system.

Clomid is another chemical drug that the medical profession praises. It is used as a fertility medicine in some women who are unable to become pregnant. It is available only with a doctor's prescription. The directions say that it is very important that your doctor check your progress at regular visits, since you must stop taking this medicine if you become pregnant. A little scary, isn't it? This medicine may cause vision problems, dizziness or lightheadedness. It has caused personality changes in some women. It is now found that some women on Clomid (another human experiment) are thrown into premature menopause.

A drug called Bendectin, which was widely prescribed for pregnancy morning sickness has been pulled off the market. It has been found to cause birth defects. The company that manufactures it is being sued. Even with all the adverse publicity the company is encouraging women who still have some not to fear taking it. A wide variety of fetal skeletal defects and other abnormalities have been reported among the offspring of mothers using this drug.

An ingredient found in hundreds of non-prescription cold remedies and sleep-aid remedies called Methapyrilene has been found to be a dangerous cancer-causing agent. The products that contain this substance include Nytol, Compoz, Sominex, Allerest and Excedrin P.M. This finding comes from the researchers at the Frederick Cancer Research Center in Maryland. Drug companies were made about the loss of business and the years of advertising, and they came out with "New Formulas" of their highly advertised products.

Dioxin has been in the news many times. Scientists estimate that if efficiently administered, an ounce of Dioxin could kill one million people. Dioxin is a byproduct of "chlorinated phenolic compounds" which serve as germ and fungus-killing agents in such products as adhesives, paints, lacquers, paper coating, wood preservatives, shampoos, and laundry starches. Dioxin has caused cancer when given to animals. It primarily affects the liver and large intestine.

Side effects are headaches, pain, excessive sweating, increased heart rates and respiratory difficulties.

Dioxin is a byproduct of hexachlorophene which used to be used in toothpastes and as an antibacterial chemical in soaps, deodorants, and vaginal aerosol sprays. In 1972, 72 French infants were dusted with talc that had accidentally been mixed with 6 percent hexachlorophene. The infants died. The FDA banned hexachlorophene, but not until millions of people had used it in all kinds of products. Hexachlorophene was used since the 1940s and it was not until the early 1970s that repeated use of this drug led to significant amounts passing into the bloodstream. It accumulates in the blood. The ironic part was this drug was shown to be ineffective. One of the investigations showed that routine bathing of infants with hexachlorophene could result in an increase of staph infections.

Valium is the most over-prescribed drug and probably the most abused drug in the United States. It has shown to produce some of the symptoms it is supposed to relieve. Many women have died in hospital emergency rooms from the misuse of tranquilizers such as valium. How many deaths are attributed to an overdose of herbs?

How many of you have heard of the DES daughters and sons? DES (diethylstilbestrol) is a hormone drug that was prescribed for women in the 50s and 60s to help prevent miscarriage. Many children born of mothers who had taken the drug are now coming down with vaginal cancer and some of the girls have had to have their vaginas replaced. Of course, they will never be able to have children. The male offspring of mothers who took the drug were found to have genitourinary defects.

DES is a synthetic sex hormone discovered in 1938. It has been injected into the necks of chickens to make them grow faster. In 1947 the Food and Drug Administration authorized its use in poultry. It was known even back then that it caused cancer in animals, and possibly in humans.

In 1954 it was approved for cattle feed. It was believed not to be in the meat when it was slaughtered, but one year later the drug residue was found in the liver, kidney and skin fat of chickens, just before they were killed. It took four years after that before it was banned in poultry, but it still wasn't banned in cattle. It was still believed the residue was not in the cattle if they withdrew the drug 48 hours before they were slaughtered. Although it was banned in 1971 for pregnant women, the population was being drugged through the beef supply. Twenty-one other nations outlawed DES. Many countries, including Sweden, refused to import beef from the U.S. because of DES. However, there are also at least 14 other hormones being fed to cattle.

There are many drugs that have caused untold misery to thousands of people. One of the worst disasters in the field of medicine took place when I was pregnant with my youngest son in 1960. In the late 1950s, sleeping pills and tranquilizers were all the rage. Mothers in 46 countries around the world, including thousands in the United States, gladly took a tranquilizing pill that was said to be safe and non-toxic for pregnant women. This wonder drug was Thalidomide. Its most terrifying side effect was missing limbs on newborn infants. Fingers and ears were missing, and cleft palate. Some had paralyzed faces, brain damage, deafness, or blindness. The truth was: eight thousand babies were horribly poisoned and entered the world with terrible deformities. It is estimated that 16 thousand died at birth, mostly from internal damage. Many hundreds of other babies suffered from faulty hearts, hearing defects and other abnormalities that have not been attributed to Thalidomide because they do not fit the most typical pattern. The sad story is told in a book called "Suffer The Children: The Story of Thalidomide."

The anguish of the parents was aggravated by the fact that many did not know that Thalidomide was to blame, because the pill was prescribed months earlier to help them sleep, relieve headaches, or quiet morning sickness. Many parents believed that something must have been wrong with them and they blamed themselves or each other for the child's deformities.

One woman had two Thalidomide children. One couple in Belgium, with the help of their family doctor, poisoned their 8 day old daughter who had been born without legs. One mistake that was made was the way malformed babies were concealed from their mothers after birth, and then suddenly presented to her with its little limbs, no limbs, or just flippers, just as they were leaving for home. The midwives and nurses made all kinds of excuses so they wouldn't have to tell them. Thousands of people suffered with this supposedly innocent drug, developed and prescribed by modern medicine.

Fathers blamed mothers and divorced them. One father told his wife that if she brought that monster home, he would leave. She brought the baby home and he left. One mother went to a hotel and committed suicide. Another mother said, "I did try to end my life. I started to take pills, but all the time I thought of her lying helpless with her awful stunted body and I keep repeating to myself, `Who would look after her?'"

The person who could have relieved some of the anguish and distress was the family doctor, but he was reluctant to speak out—partly because he felt guilty, and partly he feared the parents would sue him.

I think the medical profession should be very humble when they say that herbs are dangerous.

Of course, there are useful drugs, such as Digitalis, which have saved lives, and penicillin, which stops infections. There are times when a visit to the doctor is a wise choice; however, in most cases, the body will heal itself when given the correct diet, nutrients and herbs.

ACUTE DISEASE SYMPTOMS

Acute diseases are nature's therapy of cleansing and healing the system. The body will respond to this healing if certain rules are followed. Fasting from solid food will help nature do her job. Drinking lemon juice in pure water or herbal teas is one way to assist nature. When you stop eating solid foods, nature goes to work and cleans the cells and dumps the toxins in the stomach where they are then eliminated through the kidneys and bowels. If you keep eating when you have an acute disease, the body uses its energy to digest the food and this stops nature's natural cleansing process.

Herbs are excellent to assist nature, depending upon the symptoms the acute disease manifests. Herbal lower bowel cleanser helps to clean and restore bowel function by elimination of toxins. When we allow nature to do her job, the acute diseases will help prevent chronic diseases in the future.

The following excerpt is from a book by Henry Lindlahr, M.D., called Philosophy of Natural Therapeutics, published in 1918, which is out of print:

"From the foregoing it will have become apparent that smallpox, like every other infectious disease, is a filth disease, that its microzyma grow in morbid soil only and that the smallpox eruptions are a sign of rapid elimination of hereditary and acquired disease taints.

A good dose of smallpox may rid the system of more scrofulous, tuberculous and syphilitic poisons than could otherwise be gotten rid of in a lifetime. Therefore smallpox is certainly to be preferred to vaccination. The one means the elimination of chronic disease, the other making of it.

"Cheap talk!" someone says. Not so, my friend! This is not mere talk. I was put to the test in the case of my own family and therefore speak from personal experience. My oldest boy was born at a time when both parents were heavily encumbered with hereditary and acquired disease conditions. At birth he weighed only two and a half pounds and his chance for life seemed very slight. The eyes were of a blackish blue, especially the outer portion of the iris, and this gradually condensed into a heavy scurf rim owing to the fact that Nature's cleansing efforts in the form of skin eruptions were promptly suppressed with talcum powder and other home "remedies".

For the first five or six years of his life our boy was a weak, sickly child, having one after another all of the common infantile ailments. However, we soon learned to treat these natural methods and he was not vaccinated.

One day suspicious looking eruptions appeared, which soon spread all over his body. I called in two allopathic physicians to verify my own diagnosis of smallpox, which they did unqualifiedly.

We applied the natural treatment, which consisted of strict fasting, colon flushing and cold water applications. The child was keep day and night in wet packs—strips of linen wrung out of water of natural temperature and covered with flannel bandages—which were changed whenever they became hot and dry. The face also was kept covered with cooling compresses. In addition to this treatment I gave the indicated high potency homeopathic remedies. There was hardly a spot on the boy's body that was not covered with sores. However, constant renewal of the cold packs kept the temperature below the danger point and greatly alleviated the insufferable itching peculiar to the disease.

My wife, her sister and myself by turns slept in the same room with the child without the least fear of infection, and although we had not been vaccinated since childhood we remained unaffected by the "contagious disease".

The wet packs, of course, greatly furthered the processes of elimination, and the disease practically ran its course in ten days. From that time on the sores healed rapidly and nothing remained to indicate the "ravages" of the disease but a telltale mark over the left eyebrow and a few similar scars on the boy's body. These also have now entirely disappeared.

Under this natural treatment of the disease convalescence was rapid and complete, and soon after the eyes became much clearer and much lighter in color. Since his recovery from the smallpox this boy has never had a sick day. He is now in his twenty-first year and well developed physically and mentally.

As far as I could learn there was not another case of smallpox in Chicago and vicinity at the time of the boy's illness. If the infection theory be true, from whom did he "catch" the disease and why did not one of the many persons living in the same house become infected? My answer is: This acute eliminative process was Nature's way of purifying the little body of inherited scrofulous and other disease taints."

A faulty diet causes an accumulation of too much carbohydrates, white sugar and white flour products. The digestive system is therefore incapable of dealing with the build-up starchy waste and the tissues become clogged, constipation develops and backs up toxins and causes colds, flu, fevers and acute diseases.

Acute diseases should be taken seriously and treated naturally, otherwise they can cause further problems such as pneumonia, spinal meningitis, and strep throat.

Chiropractic-Hydrotherapy

HISTORY AND DESCRIPTION

The philosophy of chiropractic handed down since it was founded by Daniel David Palmer (in 1895) is that chiropractic is first a preventive form of health care and only secondarily a curative form. Palmer put together a synthesis of Hippocrates, Plato, Aristotle, Galen and Vesalius with a proposition which taught that (1) we should look to the spine for the cause of disease (a Hippocratic admonition) because (2) it contains and protects the spinal cord, through which vital forces flow and are mediated to all parts of the body through the spinal nerves. Therefore, chiropractic is designed to restore the normal function of the nerve system. (One chiropractor put it this way: "All I do is normalize the body.")

Every cell of your body receives nerve impulses either directly or indirectly from the spine. Each one of these large nerve cables leaving your spine carries some 300,000 tiny nerves. The therapy of chiropractic is based upon the theory that disease is caused by interference with nerve functions. The goal of chiropractic, then, is concerned with freeing the interference of bodily processes caused by blocked or damaged nerve control which render the body less resistant to infection. This is true prevention, for chiropractic attempts to enable the nervous system to perform its purposes of controlling and coordinating every cell, organ and structure in the body and to adapt the organism to its environment. The breakdown of the immunological systems and possible cancer can be avoided in the main, if the body is *free* to do what it was created to do.

Chiropractic calls these interferences *subluxations* (vertebral misalignment), and these are caused by birth, auto accidents, home accidents, practical jokes and horseplay, trauma and fear, falls, toxins from food additives, tobacco, alcohol, exhaust fumes and drugs. The subluxation is considered the main *cause* of disease, while the point at which the disease becomes apparent is the *symptom*.

TRAINING

Much of the criticism against chiropractic stems from ignorance of chiropractic training. Chiropractic students spend 4,485 hours studying many of the same things medical students (4,248 hours) study: Anatomy, Physiology, Pathology, Chemistry, Bacteriology, Diagnosis, Neurology, X-ray, Psychiatry, Orthopedics (Gynecology). Medical doctors also study Pharmacology, Immunology, and General Surgery, but since chiropractors have a different philosophy of health, they receive training in Adjusting, Manipulation, and Kinesiology instead. A student in chiropractic concentrates not on germs, but on improving the `soil conditions' of the body. He will see germs not as the prime cause of disease but as scavengers which exist to rid the body of morbid material, just as insects prey upon diseased plant life. In addition, he sees each individual patient as being biochemically unique. Yet within this uniqueness is a similarity anatomically and physiologically which enables the chiropractor to use his science.

As to those supporters of medical science who continue to call chiropractic an unscientific cult, the reader should remember that not only does the medical field espouse a different philosophy of medicine (treatment of symptoms rather than cause), it wants to have a monopoly on health care simply because it so myopically is sure that its way is the only way. Using medical bias it is certainly possible to `prove' that chiropractic is a false theory, or that educational standards are below that of MD's, or that it is dangerous. Each of these reasons has more holes in them than Swiss cheese, particularly the latter: any health care can be dangerous in the hands of he who practices not from compassion on the human condition, but simply from greed. Drug overdoses, complications from surgery, and malpractice suits are much more common among medical doctors than among any other kind of health practitioner.

TREATMENT

Although a chiropractor appears to be working primarily with the bones of your spine and skeletal system, he knows this is merely the best approach to freeing the nerves so that they may perform the natural work for which they were naturally intended. This is why some people call chiropractors nerve specialists, rather than bone doctors. The bones and skeleton are merely the keys to open the doors to the nerves.

Many chiropractors practice nutrition counseling along with their chiropractic since it has been found that a well-fed person responds to *any* helpful therapy better than the poorly-fed. Your chiropractor may supplement spinal adjustments and nutrition with electricity; water treatments; heat and cold; shoe, bed seat or work position changes; acupressure; massage; kinesiology; vitamin therapy; traction; rehabilitative exercises and, above all, a re-education into the basics of health—which MD's normally don't provide.

HYDROTHERAPY

Water is one of the best healers in existence. It is not irritating to use internally, it is good on the skin, and the only time you need to be careful is with extremes of temperatures on some people.

Water affects the entire body—muscles, nerves and liver. It can enhance the conversion of lactic acid from fatigued muscles back into useful energy. It also makes skin sensations more alive. Therapy with water can be used generally in two ways: hot or warm water and cold or cool water.

Hot or warm water dilates or expands the blood vessels that increase the speed of the blood's flow. Local application increases capillary pressure, increases the flow of fluid into the lymph spaces, increases perspiration, and relieves pain. A warm bath relieves muscle fatigue and promotes sleep and rest.

Cool or cold water when accompanied by rubbing and massage, stimulates the blood and the nerves. It begins a vascular gymnastics with the blood vessels pumping vigorously, alternating between dilation and contraction. For this reason never use cold water with exhaustion—your body won't be able to handle it. Cold delivers extra oxygen to the skin. Following a warm bath, a cold shower gives the body new energy, making the brain more alert and the extremities warmer. You will find that you will be able to accomplish more work.

There are many helpful techniques for the water to heal, soothe, stimulate or relax.

FOMENTATIONS (warm)
• relieve congestion of chest colds
• ease pain of arthritis
• stimulate (alternate with cold)
• sedate (use on spine)

HOT FOOT BATH (100-115 degrees)
• increase circulation
• heighten nerve and muscle tone, skin sensitivity
• increase antibody production

SITZ BATH
    COLD (55-75 degrees)—hemorrhoids, prostate, perinium and rectum surgery
    HOT (105-110 degrees)—treat pelvic pain during menstrual cycle, inflammatory conditions. Use cold compresses to the head and neck simultaneously.

CONTRAST BATHS (hot then cold)
• poor circulation
• arthritis

ICE PACKS
• injury, swelling, anesthetics

TUB BATHS
    Neutral (94-98 degrees)—sedative (cover the patient to the neck with a pillow under the neck)

There are other means to using water externally: epsom salts bath, sauna or steam bath, hot baths, warm baths, local wet pack, cool baths, cold baths, wet pack treatment, cold sheet treatment (Dr. Henry Lindlhar) and sulphur or pine baths. However you choose to use water as a method for improving health, Father Kneipp, the pioneer of hydrotherapy, would be proud of you for using such a simple, common technique for what ails you. And don't forget water's internal uses: douches, enemas, colonics, eye baths and mouth treatment.

SKIN BRUSHING

Regular bathing and washing will not remove the layers of dead skin. It takes a gentle and light abrasion on the skin when it is dry to rid the body of the dead unwanted skin. The dead layers need to be peeled away so the skin will be able to breathe and live properly. This is what is referred to as dry skin brushing. Acne, pimples, excessive dryness or oiliness can all be greatly helped by this activity. It increases rapid cell production beneath the surface of the skin. It is considered the same body stimulation as compared to twenty minutes jogging or fast walking. Rubbing the skin with a turkish towel will make sure the lymphatic system and bloodstream are exercised. Use a skin brush made from natural bristles, with a long but detachable handle so that you can reach your back. It is a wonderful feeling, and so stimulating to brush just before you shower. It leaves a tingling and refreshing feeling.

Skin brushing is an effective way for cleansing the lymphatic system through physically stimulating it. It also stimulates the bloodstream and is excellent for poor circulation, and is a must on a colon cleansing program. It helps to dislodge mucus in the area that is needed. Start by brushing the soles of the feet and work up each leg, up the bottom and up to the middle of the back, (avoid the genitals). Work towards the heart and bring all toxins toward the colon. Then start at the fingertips and brush up the arms, across the shoulders, down the chest and the top of the back, again avoiding sensitive parts like the nipples. Don't forget the arm pits, this is where glandular inflammation collect in the lymph. Then brush down towards the colon. On the area below the navel, brush in movements starting on the right hand side, going up, across and down, following the shape of the colon. Women should brush the breasts, it cleans and protects against lumps.

The face should always be cleaned with a wash cloth or a natural soft brush.

Another type of skin brushing or a brisk scrub is with stone ground corn meal while the skin is wet, followed by a tepid or cold rinse. This thoroughly cleanses the skin while stimulating circulation. The natural oil in the corn meals prevents irritation and leaves the skin baby soft.

Menus And Recipes

RAW FOOD DIET

*Liquids should be taken at least 30 minutes before meals.

RAW FOOD DIET

DAY I
Breakfast
Fresh sliced peaches, strawberries and bananas with nut milk
Fresh fruit juice

Lunch
Meatless Loaf
Raw vegetable juice

Dinner
Sprout Salad
(alfalfa, mung bean, lentil, radish sprouts) with romaine lettuce, radishes, cucumbers, green onions, peas
Herbed yogurt dressing
Topped with sunflower seeds
Raw carrot juice

DAY II
Breakfast
Fruit Sherbet with shredded fresh coconut

Lunch
Multi-seed Loaf
Fresh vegetable juice

Dinner
Supper Salad
Raw vegetable juice

DAY III
Breakfast
Nature's Cake
Herb tea

Lunch
Lentil Soup
Raw vegetable juice

Dinner
Total Salad
Raw vegetable juice

DAY IV
Breakfast
Apple Delight
Raw fruit juice

Lunch
Guacamole Salad Dip
Carrot sticks, celery sticks, cauliflowerettes
Raw vegetable juice

Dinner
Stuffed Peppers
Raw vegetable juice

DAY V
Breakfast
Banana Freeze
Fresh orange juice

Lunch
Cucumber Salad
Raw vegetable juice

Dinner
Corned Salad
Raw Vegetable Soup
Raw vegetable juice

DAY VI
Breakfast
Gold Salad
Raw fruit juice

Lunch
Green Soup
Raw vegetable juice

Dinner
Veggie-Fish Loaf
Raw vegetable juice

DAY VII
Breakfast
Apples Plus
Fresh fruit juice

Lunch
Cabbage Salad
Fresh vegetable juice

Dinner
Fiber Loaf
Fresh vegetable juice

RAW FOOD RECIPES

Meatless Loaf
1 c. grated carrots
1 c. diced tomatoes
1 c. chopped celery
1/4 c. diced green bell pepper
2 tblsp. salad oils
1 c. ground almonds (or enough to make a firm loaf)
Pat into oiled dish and garnish with parsley.

Fruit Sherbet
Blend orange juice, pineapple juice and diced fresh oranges and pineapple, plus one sliced banana in blender. Freeze in freezer tray. Take frozen pieces and blend with lecithin granules, 4 tblsp. honey, dash cinnamon. Serve immediately.

Multi-Seed Loaf
Soak the seeds for eight hours; drain. Grind in blender:
1 c. sunflower seeds
1 c. sesame seeds
1 c. shredded raw potato
Mix with:
1 c. shredded carrots
1 c. diced celery
1/2 c. chopped onion
1 c. diced tomato
Add enough tomato juice to moisten and mold into a loaf.

Supper Salad
dressing: plain yogurt, paprika, ground dill
2 Jerusalem artichokes, sliced thinly
2 Tblsp. chopped green onion
Dash of kelp
Red onion, separated into rings
1 small bunch of radishes, sliced
watercress, rinsed and chopped
torn salad greens (red leaf, beet greens)
1 sliced avocado
1 med. sliced tomato
1/2 cucumber, sliced
1 small green pepper, chopped
Lightly toss all vegetables together. Serve with dressing.

Nature's Cake
1 c. rolled oats
1 c. ground almonds
1 tsp. cinnamon
1/2 tsp. nutmeg
1/4 tsp. cloves
1/2 c. unsweetened shredded coconut
1/4 c. honey
3 Tblsp. apple juice
3 Tblsp. raw applesauce
1/2 c. tahini (almond paste)
1 c. raisins
1/2 c. ground dates
3 c. shredded carrots
Grind the raisins, dates and carrots together and add to honey, apple juice and
applesauce. Mix in tahini and dry ingredients. Pat into a loaf pan and refrigerate
at least 2 hours.

Lentil Soup
2 c. sprouted lentils
1 med. potato, chopped
1/2 c. chopped parsley
1/2 c. chopped celery
2 c. grated zucchini
1/4 c. chopped onion
Blend in blender. Heat and serve with dollop of plain yogurt.

Total Salad
1 c. mung bean sprouts
1 c. alfalfa sprouts
1/2 avocado, sliced
sliced tomato, cucumber, radishes
1/2 c. sliced zucchini
1 sm. sliced bell pepper
1/2 c. sliced green onions
Mixed salad (dark) greens
Toss all together. Serve with fresh lemon squeezed over all. Garnish with sunflower seeds.

Apple Delight
2 large apples, grated
1/4 c. raisins, ground
1/4 c. dates, ground
1/2 c. sunflower seeds, ground
1/2 c. apple juice
dash cinnamon
1 Tblsp. honey
Mix together, chill and serve.

Guacamole
2 medium avocados, mashed
1 large peeled tomato, chopped
1 T. red minced onion
1 T. fresh parsley
1 T. fresh lemon juice
Kelp to taste
Mix all ingredients together and serve on a bed of fresh greens. Use as a dip with fresh vegetables.

Stuffed Peppers

2 large green peppers, cut in half
Mix together:
1/2 c. celery, chopped
1 tomato, chopped
3 green onions, chopped
1 c. fresh peas
1/4 c. ground almonds
homemade mayonnaise to moisten
Prepare green peppers and chill in cold water for a few hours. Mix all other
ingredients together and fill the green pepper halves just before ready to eat.

Banana Freeze

Blend 3 bananas in blender, with 1 tsp. fresh lemon juice and 1/4 tsp. cardamon,
with 2 Tblsp. honey. Freeze in trays.
*Can be eaten fresh, without freezing.

Cool Salad

This is a basic, raw food recipe.
1 large sliced cucumber
3 large tomatoes, chopped
1 red pepper, chopped
1 c. mung bean sprouts
1/4 c. chopped raw cashews
1/4 lemon, juiced
2 T. chopped green onion
Vegetable seasoning to taste.

Raw Carrot Soup

1 c. carrot juice
1/2 lemon, juiced
1 tsp. olive oil
1 clove garlic
Blend, then mix in:
1/2 c. chopped tomato
1 tsp. chopped onion
1/2 c. grated celery
1/4 c. chopped red bell pepper

Corned Salad

4 ears sweet corn, scraped
1 c. diced, ripe tomato
1 c. shredded yellow crookneck squash
2 Tblsp. chopped green onion
2 Tblsp. chopped bell pepper
1/4 tsp. dill
1/4 tsp. marjoram
1/4 tsp. paprika
1 c. alfalfa sprouts
Mix together and serve with favorite dressing.

Gold Salad

1/2 c. soaked dried apricots
2 Tbsp. shredded fresh coconut
1 c. red seedless grapes
1 sliced banana
1 chopped ripe pear
2 Tbsp. almonds
Mix together and serve.

Green Soup

1 bunch green onions, chopped
2 c. shredded savoy cabbage
1 avocado
4 c. water
1 tsp. vegetable seasoning
1/4 tsp. cayenne pepper
Blend all vegetables in a small amount of water, gradually adding 4 cups of
water. Add veg. seasonings and cayenne pepper.

Vegetable Loaf

1/2 c. chopped almonds
1 c. carrot pulp
2 stalks celery
1 c. chopped green onions
Fresh or dried basil
1/8 c. rejuvelac or water
1 c. sesame seeds
1/4 bunch finely chopped parsley
1 green pepper, minced
dill weed to taste
vegetable seasoning to taste
Grind almonds and seeds and add carrots, parsley, and remaining ingredients.
Mix with hands. If too thick, add more water, a little at a time. Place in a dish
and refrigerate for 6-8 hours.

Apples Plus
Six apples
2 bananas, diced
3 peaches, diced
2 pears, diced
Dig out the centers of apples, about 3/4 of way down. Add the apple pulp to rest of fruit, minus the seeds, core and membranes. Fill the apples with fruit stuffing and sprinkle with grated almonds.

Cabbage Salad
1 c. red cabbage, chopped
1 c. savoy cabbage, chopped
1/2 c. chopped celery
1 c. chopped red onion
1 c. coarsely chopped pecans
Leaf lettuce
Olive oil
Lemon juice
Mix all together and add equal parts olive oil and lemon juice. Serve on lettuce leaves.

Fiber Loaf
2 c. ground sesame seeds
4 c. ground sunflower seeds
10 lg. mushrooms, chopped
1 c. diced parsley
3 cloves garlic, finely chopped
4 stalks celery, finely diced
pinch of sweet basil
1/2 tsp. dill
Vegetable seasoning to taste
Mix ground seeds together. Add enough water or rejuvelac so that the ground seeds stick together. Add diced vegetables and seasonings, according to taste. Place in warm place 12-24 hours, (70 degrees to 90 degrees), until top is firm.

COOKED FOOD DIET

DAY I
Breakfast
Fruit Salad
Steamed millet (thermos method)

Lunch
Wild Rice Medley
Cheese Enchiladas
Green Salad

Dinner
Yam Bake
Soup of the Day

DAY II
<u>Breakfast</u>
Apple Salad

<u>Lunch</u>
Steamed broccoli
Baked potato with yogurt and chopped green onions
Whole grain roll

Dinner
Vegetable Chop Suey
Steamed brown rice
Green salad

DAY III
<u>Breakfast</u>
Super Breakfast Cereal
Juice

<u>Lunch</u>
Pinto Bean Stew
Green Salad

<u>Dinner</u>
Strawberry Jell Salad

DAY IV
<u>Breakfast</u>
Glazed Fresh Fruit
Steamed whole oats

<u>Lunch</u>
Spanish Millet Loaf
Whole grain roll

<u>Dinner</u>
Potato Salad
Green Salad

DAY V
<u>Breakfast</u>
Steamed wheat berries (thermos method)
Sliced peaches or other fruit in season

<u>Lunch</u>
Lima Bean Casserole
Chapatis
Vegetable juice

<u>Dinner</u>
Barley Salad
Whole grain roll

DAY VI
<u>Breakfast</u>
Nut and Seed Granola
Sliced fruit in season

<u>Lunch</u>
Spaghetti Squash w/tomato sauce and Italian herb seasoning
Steamed brown rice

<u>Dinner</u>
Navy Bean Soup
Whole grain roll
Vegetable juice

DAY VII
<u>Breakfast</u>
Fresh, sliced fruit in season with yogurt dressing
(Plain yogurt, fresh lemon juice, honey and cinnamon to taste)

<u>Lunch</u>
Rice, Mexican Style
Vegetable juice

<u>Dinner</u>
Summer Salad

COOKED FOOD RECIPES

Wild Rice Medley
1/2 c. wild rice
1/2 c. Basmate rice
1/4 c. olive oil
1/2 onion, chopped
1/2 green pepper, chopped
1/4 c. chopped almonds
2 Tblsp. lemon juice
Heat 3 cups water to boiling. Add rice. Cook (covered) for 30 minutes. Turn off heat. Let pan sit for 20 minutes with lid on. This will finish steam-cooking it. Turn into bowl. Toss with rest of ingredients. Add seasonings to taste.

Cheese Enchiladas
12 corn tortillas
2 c. mild cheese, grated
1/2 c. onion, chopped
1 small can diced green chiles
1 tall can enchilada sauce
1 small can tomato sauce
1 pint sour cream or mock sour cream
Black olives (optional) to sprinkle on top
Heat enchilada sauce and tomato sauce and add 1 small can of water. Mix the cheese, onions and chiles. Dip tortilla in the hot sauce mix to soften. Place about 2 T. of the cheese mixture on tortilla; top with a heaping tablespoon of sour cream; roll the tortilla and place seam side down and put in a baking dish. When all tortillas are rolled up, pour the rest of the enchilada sauce on the top and sprinkle top with cheese and olives. Bake in a 350 degree F. oven for about 30 minutes.

Yam Bake
2 c. mashed, cooked yams or sweet potatoes
1 c. ripe mashed banana
1/3 c. yogurt or sour cream
1 egg
1/2 tsp. mineral salt
2 T. pure maple syrup or honey
Blend all ingredients together. Beat until smooth. Bake in a buttered casserole dish at 350 degrees for 20 minutes. Serves 4 to 6.

Soup of the Day
Bring to boil:
2 quarts water
1 teaspoon salt
1 teaspoon garlic powder
2 teaspoons chopped basil
2 small cans tomato sauce
Turn down heat and add sliced carrots, celery, cooked whole grain (rice or millet) in any quantity you desire. Simmer for 20 minutes.

Apple Salad
3 apples, cored and chopped
2 stalks celery, chopped
1 cup walnuts, chopped
Salad dressing to moisten. Toss all ingredients together. Chill and serve.

Vegetable Chop Suey
1 c. green and red peppers, sliced diagonally
1 c. celery, sliced diagonally
1/2 c. onions, sliced
1 small can water chestnuts, sliced
1 c. bamboo shoots
1 c. mung bean sprouts
1 c. mushrooms, sliced
1/8 tsp. ginger
2 cloves garlic, minced
4 T. butter
4 tsp. tamari (soy sauce)
1 T. sesame seeds
Cook vegetables lightly and serve over cooked brown rice or millet. Vegetables should be crunchy.

Super Breakfast Cereal
1/2 c. oatmeal
1 c. plain yogurt
2 T. orange juice
1 T. honey
1/2 c. raisins
1/4 c. almonds, chopped
1 T. sesame seeds
1/2 c. chopped peaches
1/2 c. chopped apples
1/2 c. sliced bananas
Fold all ingredients together. You can substitute sunflower seeds for sesame seeds, pecans for almonds.

Strawberry Jell Salad
2 c. fruit and berry juice (frozen)
3 T. agar-agar flakes
3 T. honey
2 c. strawberries, sliced
2 bananas, sliced
1 T. fresh lemon juice
Dissolve agar-agar in the juice by bringing to a boil and simmer on low for about 5 minutes. Cool, add the strawberries, bananas, honey and lemon juice. Chill in a mold. Serves 6.

Pinto Bean Stew
2 c. pinto beans, cooked
4 c. vegetable broth
1 c. carrots, sliced
1/2 c. broccoli, sliced
1/2 c. zucchini
1/2 c. celery, sliced
3 large tomatoes, peeled and chopped
2 T. olive oil
1 T. vegetable seasoning
1 T. kelp
Sauté onions and garlic in oil in a large stew pan. Add all ingredients and water if needed. Bring to a boil, reduce heat and simmer about 15 minutes, until vegetables are still crunchy.

Glazed Fresh Fruit
1 c. fruit and berry juice, unsweetened (frozen section)
1 T. arrowroot or cornstarch
1/4 tsp. ginger
1/2 tsp. cardamon
2 c. fresh strawberries
1 c. apples, chopped
1 c. seedless grapes, halved
1 c. fresh peaches, sliced
Stir arrowroot and seasonings in juice over stove and bring to a boil; cook for one minute. Toss fruit together and fold in juice mixture and stir to coat well. Chill. Serves 6.

Spanish Millet Loaf
2 c. cooked millet
1 c. whole wheat bread crumbs
1 small can green chiles
1 c. canned tomatoes
2 beaten eggs
2 T. vegetable seasoning
1 c. ground almonds
2 T. olive oil
1 tsp. chili powder
Combine all ingredients together. Pour into a buttered loaf pan. Cook for 45 minutes at 350 degrees F. While cooking, baste with butter two or three times. It may be served with uncooked salsa.

Potato Soup
4 large potatoes
3 c. water
2 T. raw cashew butter
1 small onion
4 stalks celery, chopped
1/2 c. freshly chopped parsley
1 tsp. vegetable salt
Steam potatoes with skins on in the water. Remove skin from potatoes and mash through dicer. Dissolve nut butter in 1 c. of warm pure water. Put all other ingredients together and cook in double boiler for about 20 minutes.

Lima Bean Casserole
4 c. cooked fresh lima beans
1 c. finely chopped onions
2 cloves garlic, minced
1/2 tsp. kelp
1 grated carrot
2 stalks chopped celery
1 Tbsp. chopped red or green pepper
1 tsp. Italian mixed herbs
2 Tbsp. tomato paste
2 Tbsp. butter or olive oil
Put beans in a baking dish. Add all ingredients except juice and butter. Stir well. Add tomato paste and mix with beans. Pour melted butter or olive oil over top. Bake 1 hour at 350 degree F. oven. Serves 6-8.

Chapatis
1 1/2 c. whole wheat pastry flour
1/2 c. water—more if needed
1 T. cold pressed oil
Mix the flour, water and oil. Knead the dough until it is smooth and elastic.
Pinch off the dough into balls. Should make about eight. Flatten the dough in the
palm of your hand and roll it out on a floured surface into a circle about seven
inches in diameter. Use an iron or stainless heavy griddle. Cook each side until
brown. Needs to be a hot pan and will dry out if it is not hot enough. Keep pan
clean from burned flour before cooking another.

Barley Salad
1 2/3 c. vegetable broth
1 c. whole barley, rinsed
1 c. grated carrots
1/2 c. sliced radishes
1/4 c. chopped fresh parsley
1 1/3 c. water
1/2 c. chopped green pepper
1/2 c. chopped red pepper
1/2 c. chopped Bermuda onion
1 Tbsp. dried dillweed

Salad Dressing
1 pressed clove of garlic
1/2 tsp. vegetable seasoning
1/4 tsp. white pepper
2 Tbsp. olive oil
3 Tbsp. fresh lemon juice
Bring water and broth to a boil, then add barley. Reduce heat, cover pan and
simmer the barley for about an hour, or until done. Mix all dressing ingredients
in a bowl. Add cooked barley to dressing while it is still warm. Mix all
ingredients well except the vegetables, which you can add and toss well just
before serving.

Nut and Seed Granola
1 c. ground sunflower seeds
1 c. ground sesame seeds
1/8 c. ground chia seeds
1/8 c. ground flax seeds
1 c. freshly grated coconut
1 c. ground almonds
1 1/2 t. grated orange rind
1/2 t. cardamon
1/2 c. date sugar
1/2 c. warm honey
Mix all together and drip warm honey and stir. Keep in a tight jar in a cool place.
Can cook in the oven at 200 degrees F. for about an hour, stirring often.

Navy Bean Soup
2 c. navy beans
8 c. vegetable broth
1 c. sliced carrots
2 stalks celery, chopped
1 onion, minced
2 tsp. salt
Dash of herbs of choice (basil, mixed Italian, etc.)
Wash beans and soak in water overnight. Add soaked beans to boiling vegetable
broth. Reduce heat and cook on low for an hour or until done. Add vegetables
and herbs and cook until vegetables are still crunchy (about 15 minutes). Serve
with plain yogurt and parsley on top.

Fruit Dip Dressing
Plain yogurt
lemon juice
honey
cinnamon
Mix to taste. Serve with apple wedges, grapes, banana chunks or strawberries.

Rice Mexican Style

5 c. cooked brown rice
1 med. onion, diced
1/2 c. green pepper, diced
1/2 c. red pepper, diced
1/2 c. chopped green onions
1 c. mushrooms, sliced
2 cloves of garlic, pressed
1/4 c. canned green chilies
2 c. canned peeled tomatoes, chopped (and juice)
1/4 c. sliced black olives
2 tsp. chili powder
1 tsp. ground cumin
dash of hot sauce
Sauté the onions, peppers, green onions and garlic lightly in one tablespoon of olive oil for a few minutes. Add mushrooms and sauté a few minutes longer. Then add all remaining ingredients, stir, then cook five to ten minutes until it is heated thoroughly. Serve the vegetables over the rice.

Summer Salad

1 c. fresh peas
4 carrots, thinly sliced
3 celery stalks, thinly sliced
6 radishes, sliced
1 green pepper, thinly sliced
6 green onions with stems
2 ears corn, cut off cob
4 c. cooked new potatoes, diced
1 c. lightly steamed green beans
Boston lettuce leaves
3 large tomatoes, cut in thin slices
Add all ingredients together, except the tomatoes. Chill in refrigerator. Toss all ingredients with herb vinaigrette dressing. Add kelp to taste. Arrange mixture into salad bowl, lined with washed lettuce leaves. Garnish with sliced tomatoes, and sunflower seeds, if desired. Add vegetable seasoning or kelp to taste.

THERMOS COOKING

Thermos cooking is an excellent way to supply nutrients to the body that are lacking in the typical American diet. Cooking in a thermos is a long slow gentle way to use grains without destroying the B-complex vitamins and enzymes, as well as vitamins. High heat cooking is destructive to whole grains.

A wide-mouthed thermos is ideal. It makes the food easier to remove. You rinse the thermos first with boiling water and spoon in the rinsed grain. Then fill to the top with boiling water, close the lid tightly and leave to cook overnight.

There will be plenty of water-space to take care of expansion. Use the extra juice to drink, it is full of enzymes and vitamins and will be healing for the digestive tract.

For grains use 1/2 cup to 1 and 1/2 cups of boiling water. This works well for a pint thermos. Wash the grain well and drain off water. Put the grain in the thermos and to scald the grain pour in boiling water and leave a few minutes to heat both the grain and the thermos. Drain again, and leave the grain in the thermos. Fill to the top with boiling water, close the thermos tightly and leave 12 hours (overnight) for most varieties of grains.

MIXED GRAINS: Mix the following grains: Buckwheat, Whole Oats, Hard Wheat, Rye and Whole Barley. Use 1/2 cup of this mixture with 1 1/2 cup of boiling water.

WHOLE WHEAT: Use 1/2 cup wheat to 1 and 1/2 cups water. For a quart thermos use 1 cup of wheat to 3 cups of water. The results are excellent using the directions above.

BROWN RICE: A nice treat for breakfast. Use 1/2 cup to a pint thermos to 1 and 1/2 cups boiling water.

BUCKWHEAT: Use 1/2 cup buckwheat groats to 1 1/2 cups water. It takes only two hours in the thermos to cook. But leave it overnight for a morning treat.

BARLEY: Use 1/2 cup barley and use the method above. It will cook in 12 hours.

MILLET: This cereal needs to be brought to the boiling point and simmered for five minutes before putting in the thermos or the hard hulls will not be broken.

Millet is an alkaline cereal and is easily assimilated and digested. Cook it half and half with brown rice.

Acute And Chronic Ailments

"Our present system recognizes disease only when it has reached crisis proportions. This is tantamount to saying that a fire is fire when it has burst through the roof, when in actuality, it was a fire when the cigarette butt began to smolder in the rug"

Carlton Fredericks

ABSCESS

Includes boils, carbuncles (a large boil with multiple heads), felon or whitlow. A boil on the edge of the eye is called a sty. An abscess is a localized, inflamed area due to infection. It has an accumulation of white, yellow or green pus. It is nature's way of isolating, cleaning and eliminating infections. They are usually found just beneath the skin, although they can be found anywhere, such as in the brain, lungs, gums, teeth, ears, tonsils, sinuses, breasts, kidneys or in any part of the body. Boils start as a raised patch of skin, then turn red or purple, and become swollen and painful. An imbalance in the body can cause boils. Impure blood and poor fat metabolism is one cause. Frequent recurring boils may indicate problems such as diabetes.

The skin is the body's largest elimination organ. It is eliminating acids, gases, vapors and toxins constantly. When the skin becomes congested it usually caused from toxins in the urinary tract. Skin problems and urinary tract infections go hand in hand.

People who have skin problems will usually have kidney and bladder problems. The filtering system of the kidneys become clogged with built-up mucus,and needs to be dissolved for better elimination.

Boils can spread when the pus is draining, be sure and sterilize anything that comes in contact with them, especially clothing. Merely washing them is insufficient.

Dr. Robert S. Mendelsohn said that the most common cause of rectal abscess in babies is severe constipation. This goes along with the skin trying to eliminate when the kidneys and colon are congested. Babies can be born with poor colon function.

NATURAL THERAPY—Cleansing the blood and using natural, herbal anti-biotics. A lower bowel cleanser will speed up the removal of toxins, juice fasts, eating a lot of fresh salads; stay with the alkaline foods.

External—Slippery elm,black walnut and fenugreek poultice in a powdered form, moistened with aloe vera juice or pure water. Apply externally to help dissolve abscesses and boils. Lemon juice applied externally and taken internally with pure water. A poultice made with charcoal and water will help draw out the poisons. Use a clean piece of cotton.

FOODS TO HEAL—Vegetables and fruits, raw and lightly steamed. Fresh vegetable juices (carrot, celery), Vegetable green drinks. Citrus fruits and juices are cleansing, (limes, lemons, oranges and grapefruit). Carrots, apricots, parsley, sprouts, yellow fruits and vegetables, cherries, green peppers, broccoli, red cabbage, berries, papaya, asparagus, leaf lettuce, pineapple, sweet potatoes, winter squash, oats, millet, brown rice, sesame seeds, blackstrap molasses, almonds, pumpkin seeds, barley, potatoes, yams.

VITAMINS AND MINERALS—Vita. in A (large amounts for a week), B Complex vitamins (speeds healing), C (with bioflavonoids, speeds healing), E (ip to 800 I.U. a day, use externally to prevent scarring). MINERALS—Multi-mineral, extra calcium and magnesium balance, manganese, silicon, selenium and zinc(50 to 100 mg. per day), it is very healing.

HERBAL COMBINATIONS—Blood purifier, Antibiotic and Lower Bowel formulas. External: Black herbal ointment, or a Golden Seal ointment.

SINGLE HERBS—Aloe Vera (heals scar tissue, boils leave scars), Burdock (antibiotic and blood cleanser), Black Walnut, Capsicum, Chaparral, Echinacea (heals and cleans blood), Garlic (natural antibiotic), Ginger, Golden Seal, (antiseptic, and antibiotic), Horsetail, Kelp, Marshmallow (use internally and as a poultice) Myrrh, Pau D'Arco, Parsley, Plantain (soothes inflammation and heals scar tissues), Red Clover (blood purifier), Slippery Elm (contains demulcent properties, healing), Yarrow, Yellow Dock.

SUPPLEMENTS—Acidophilus, Bee Pollen, Blue-green algae (increases oxygen utilization and protects against viral infections), Liquid Chlorophyll, Flaxseed Poultice and Clay Packs, Chinese Essential Formula, Tea Tree Oil. Essential Fatty Acids such as: Salmon Oil, Evening Primrose Oil (protects the immune system).

AVOID—Sugar, and all sugar products. White flour and pastry, Meat, cheese, Fried foods. Antibiotics (weakens the immune system). Avoid a high fat diet, chocolate, pastries, candy, cookies, ice cream and all soft drinks.

ADDICTIONS

Addiction may be mental or emotional. We may suspect addictions when there are repeated foods or substances we feel our body has to have at all times. Sugar is the underlying basis for most addictions. It gives us (false) energy. Mental work requires a lot of energy. We can add more fresh or dried fruits, for more mental work. Industry puts sugar in almost all food. The following can be addictive: Alcohol, coffee, tea, drugs, sugar, tobacco, chocolate, illegal drugs, over-the-counter drugs, caffeine drinks, and prescribed drugs.

Addictions are damaging to the brain, nervous system, digestion, liver and pancreas. Alcohol and drugs destroy brain cells and weaken the hypothalamus (appetite control), creating a craving or addiction. The immune system is affected and it leaves the body open to all kinds of diseases.

Addictions depletes the essential vitamins and minerals, while giving a false sense of energy. Excessive liquids eliminate minerals from the body as well as the B-complex vitamins. Junk food increases the body's dependency on addictions. Junk food does not satisfy the body's need for nutrients. Hypoglycemia is very often linked with addictions.

NATURAL THERAPY—Cleansing the blood and strengthening the liver, digestion, and the nerves. Juice fast using carrot, celery, parsley, as well as green drinks. Fresh apple juice. Skin brushing with hot and cold showers will cause sweating to help clean out the toxins. Steamed vegetables provide minerals to the body. Use pure water, vegetables broths and a lot of fruit and vegetable salads.

FOODS TO HEAL—Yellow fruits and vegetables, green leafy vegetables. Vegetable juices. Grains (thermos cooking to retain the B-complex vitamins and enzymes). Wheatgrass juice is healing. Those who have been heavy meat eaters can substitute meat with grains. Buckwheat, millet, brown rice, whole oats, wheat, and barley. Beans are nourishing. Nuts, seeds and sprouts of all kinds will help supply the body natural nutrients. Roasted grain drinks help in coffee addictions. A balanced diet will satisfy the body's need and help control addictions.

VITAMINS AND MINERALS—Vitamin A, (strengthens the immune system, protects the lungs), B-Complex (calms the nerves), C (cleanser and healer). Calcium (calming for the nerves), selenium, Zinc (depleted in addictions). Multi-mineral supplement to strengthen the whole body.

HERBAL COMBINATIONS—Digestion, Glands, Heart, Liver and Nerves.

SINGLE HERBS—Alfalfa (balances body, supplies minerals), Black Cohosh, Black Walnut, Burdock (purifies the blood), Capsicum, Chaparral, Dandelion (protects and nourishes the liver), Echinacea (clean the lymphatics and blood), Garlic, Gentian (cleans and heals the digestive system), Ginger, Ginkgo (strengthens the whole body), Golden Seal (healing and purifying), Gotu Kola (strengthens the brain), Hawthorn (improves heart function), Ho Sho-Wu (improves energy output), Hops (builds the nerves), Kelp, Licorice, Lobelia, Milk Thistle, Pau D'Arco, Passion Flower, Red Clover (cleans the blood and liver), Saffron (helps in digestion of fats), Scullcap, Valerian, Wood Betony.

SUPPLEMENTS—Evening Primrose Oil, Salmon Oil, Rice Bran Syrup,

Liquid Chlorophyll, herbal Teas (rich in minerals), use teas that contain nervine herbs (chamomile, hops, scullcap, catnip). Grain Drinks (substitute for coffee.)

AVOID—Sugar (increases addictions), try to eliminate meat if possible, especially beef (accumulates hormones, antibiotics, and uric acid in the body). Avoid all food and drugs that may cause a dependency. Nicotine, alcohol, caffeine, marijuana, cocaine are all habit forming. Caffeine and sugar together are addictive (they give a false sense of energy).

AGING

Aging is a natural process that gradually develops from the time you are born. It's a state that is usually arrived at slowly but life stresses can determine an early aging process.   Premature aging can develop with constant sickness, exhaustion and stresses of life.

Although we cannot avoid aging we can control the diseases that accompany old age. Chronological age is determined by years of existence. Physical or biological age is determined by functional activity and is a true indicator of true age and quality of life.

The thymus gland shrinks under stress, and it is the master gland of the immune system. The nutrients that nourish the thymus are essential to longevity and health. Lifestyle change in the areas of diet and exercise can add years to your life as well as increase happiness through good health. It doesn't matter how long you live as long as you are happy and healthy.

Use correct food combining for proper nutrition. Eat less food, but choose it wisely. A single nutrient deficiency can result in a faulty immune system, and determine our response to disease.

The happiest and most active elderly Americans are the ones that eat healthy and have more mental and physical energy.

NATURAL THERAPY—Keeping the blood clean, the bowels open and the glands fed. Exercise physically as well as mentally. A positive attitude protects the immune system. Increased supplements are needed along with digestive enzymes and hydrochloric acid to assure assimilation of supplements and food.

FOODS TO HEAL—High quality Protein and amino acids (soy milk drinks), Millet and buckwheat contain protein, raw vegetables, fruits, grains, seeds, nuts and sprouts. Broccoli, cabbage, cauliflower, and eat a lot of fiber foods (psyllium). Cut down on fats and sugar products.

VITAMINS AND MINERALS—Vitamins A, C, and E along with mineral selenium are all natural antioxidants and destroy free radicals, and protects against toxins, viruses and bacteria, smog and radiation. Vitamin D increases absorption of minerals in the bones and calcium from the stomach. B-complex (deficiencies are seen in the elderly), especially B-6, pantothenic acid , folic acid and B-12. Vitamin C, (essential for the production of interferon, that destroys viruses), it protects cells and heals wounds. Vitamin E, increases resistance to disease. Selenium protects against cancer and improves antibody production.

   Zinc builds the immune system, and is healing for wounds. All vitamins and minerals work together. Calcium can be obtained from an herbal calcium formula. Minerals from herbs such as alfalfa, kelp and dulse.

HERBAL COMBINATIONS—Bone, Chelation formula, (cleans the veins), Digestion, Endurance, Glands and Immune combinations.

SINGLE HERBS—Alfalfa, Cayenne, Damiana, Dong Quai (strengthens all female organs), Eyebright (cleans and protects the eyes), False Unicorn, Garlic (protects the veins and immune system), Gentian, Ginkgo (strengthens blood vessels, increases blood flow to brain), Ginseng (strengthens whole body, prevents senility), Gotu Kola (improves memory and brain function), Hawthorn (builds heart muscles and dilates blood vessels), Hops, Horsetail, (calcium), Ho Shou-Wu (improves health, stamina), Kelp (chelates metals), Lady's Slipper, Licorice (increases energy), Lobelia, Oatstraw, Papaya, Pau D'Arco, Red Clover, Sarsaparilla, Suma (immune system booster), Yellow Dock (rich in plant iron), Yucca (cleans deep in the cells).

SUPPLEMENTS—Bee Pollen and Spirulina (RNA-DNA), Evening Primrose Oil, Fish Oil Lipids, Salmon Oil, Lecithin (choline and inositol), Royal Jelly (dilates and strengthens the blood vessels, tissue rebuilder, and feed the glands), Whey powder (help joints remain limber and prevents calcium deposits), Blue-green algae (provides oxygen to the cells and builds the immune system).

AVOID—Processed foods, coffee, tea, cocoa, caffeine drinks. Alcohol (dilates the blood vessels and causes weak veins). Excessive consumption of soft drinks can deplete calcium, because of its high content of phosphorus. Increases bone problems such as osteoporosis. Chlorinated water speeds the aging process. Avoid salt, fats and sugar. Also avoid tobacco, red meat, alcohol, coffee, tea and caffeine drinks.

AIDS

(Acquired Immune Deficiency Syndrome)

With this disease, the immune system is completely broken down by a virus, and is complicated by other disorders which accompany it. This is indeed a modern day plague. The immune system must be rejuvenated and healed. Dr. Eva Snead, M.D. did extensive research on AIDS and discovered that some viral vaccines are made from the kidney of the African Green Monkey. She said that the African Green monkey contains hundreds of viruses, and the monkey cells are loaded with the AIDS virus. She discovered that the virus was developed in a laboratory from the kidney of the African Green Monkey, and that the World Health Organization (WHO) had "triggered" the AIDS epidemic in Africa through the WHO smallpox immunization program. The WHO vaccinated 37 million in Zaire, 19 million in Zambia, 15 million in Tanzania, 12 million in Uganda and 8 million in Malawi. It is estimated that one third of the African population could have the disease within the next six years.

The mass majority of people in 'he world get immunized, about four billion, along with booster shots. Why is Africa harboring AIDS? Could there be a connection between vaccinations and AIDS?

In Dr. Douglasses book, "AIDS, The End Of Civilization", he calls AIDS, The Greatest Biological Disaster In The History Of Mankind. I am inclined to believe these doctors. We are seeing too many people with AIDS, and other immune related diseases. Dr. Snead said that everyone who has been vaccinated has the AIDS virus in them as well as forty other viruses, including the Epstein Barr virus.

Dr. Eva Snead realized in her research that the AIDS virus has the same symptoms, in the last stages, as T-cell Leukemia. It is caused by a virus. The symptoms of T-cell Leukemia are low grade fever, enlarged lymph glands, immune deficiency, weakness, aches and pains, total loss of energy,bone pain and many other symptoms. It is very interesting that the symptoms of T-cell Leukemia are the same symptoms as many other diseases including AIDS and Epstein-Barr virus syndrome. Could it be that AIDS is a new name given to an old disease, T-cell Leukemia?

FOODS TO HEAL—80% raw food diet (raw fruits and vegetables, especially foods high in vitamins A and C which are: Fish liver oils, yellow vegetables and fruits, citrus fruits, strawberries, kale, alfalfa sprouts, papaya, broccoli, parsley and wheatgrass).

Onions, garlic, cabbage, turnips, winter squash. Use kelp and paprika and herbs for seasoning, along with fresh lemon juice and cold-pressed oils. Use millet or rice cakes instead of bread. Use millet, brown rice, buckwheat and wild rice dishes. Sprouts will provide live enzymes to help supply nutrients.

VITAMINS AND MINERALS—Multivitamins with extra A, B-complex, C with bioflavonoids, D, and E (build up the immune system).

Multi-minerals with extra calcium (an herbal calcium will supply silicon for calcium assimilation), selenium and zinc.

HERBAL COMBINATIONS—Blood Purifier, Digestion, Infection, Immune, Liver, Lower Bowels and Nerve formulas. A Garlic Anti-Plague formula will protect and build the immune system.

SINGLE HERBS—Black Walnut (expels worms and balances minerals), Burdock (cleans the blood), Cayenne, Chaparral (cleans deep into the cells), Echinacea (cleans the lymphatics for pure blood), Garlic (a natural antibiotic), Golden Seal (cleans the digestive system for better assimilation), Kelp, Marshmallow, Milk Thistle (heals and restores liver function), Pau D'Arco (cleans blood and protects the liver), Red Clover (blood purifier), Sarsaparilla, Scullcap, Suma (strengthens the whole body), Wormwood.

SUPPLEMENTS—Acidophilus, Algin, Bee Pollen, Caprylic Acid, Evening Primrose oil, Lecithin, Spirulina, Wheat Grass juice, Green drinks, Chlorophyll. Digestive Enzymes and Hydrochloric Acid tablets to help in digestion and assimilation.

AVOID—Processed foods, salt, processed meats (bacon, hot dogs, etc), white sugar, white flour, excessive dairy products (eggs, cheese, pasteurized milk). Avoid all pickled products: salad dressings, green olives, relishes. All dry roasted nuts. Avoid potato chips, pretzels, crackers, soda pop, bacon, salt pork, lunch meats and cheeses of all kinds. Avoid leftover food, where molds and yeast grow and thrive.

ALLERGIES

Digestion problems and a faulty immune system can precipitate allergic reactions in the body. The body is sensitive and reacts to certain irritants, which otherwise would not affect it. Allergic symptoms can range from the common hayfever type (sneezing, red eyes) to fatigue, irritability and myriads of other symptoms. An easy way to determine if you have a food allergy is to relax. Then take the pulse of your wrist for sixty seconds. Record the number of beats. Then eat the food you think you may be allergic to. After 15-20 minutes take your pulse again. If it increases more than ten beats per minute, you can suspect an allergy. Refrain from eating that food for one month, then eat it and test again. A average pulse reading is 52-70. You can also determine allergies by muscle-testing.

Causes of allergies are poor diet, with digestion and assimilation problems, with toxins being absorbed into the blood and lymphatic system, causing excess mucus. The excess mucus can be secreted in different areas of the body such as the nasal passages, bronchials, lungs, ears, eyes, or in the reproductive organs causing whitish or clear discharge. For more information read "Allergies: A Nutritional Approach" by Louise Tenney.

Undigested proteins act as irritants in the body. The cells treat them as foreign invaders, thus inviting an "allergic attack." An efficient digestive system is necessary to prevent accumulations of these substances in the bloodstream. Mucous membranes line many areas of the body—nose, throat, most organs and glands and the gastrointestinal tract. Healthy mucous membranes will not allow the undigested proteins to enter the bloodstream.

The colon, which is the "intestinal" part of the system, plays a vital function in preventing allergies. Its role is to eliminate waste material. However, due to faulty eating habits, eating junk food, wrong combination of foods, too much meat and an unbalanced diet, the colon becomes congested or "constipated." It will then harbor all manner of toxins, which will poison the body when released into the blood stream. This state of autointoxication lowers immune capability of the body and sets the stage or condition for allergies to occur.

NATURAL THERAPY—Blood purification and a cleansing diet. Digestion of food must be complete (food enzymes and hydrochloric acid), and the bowels must be kept clean. Juice fasts using carrot, celery and raw apple juice. Liver cleanse: when the liver is clogged with fats and accumulated toxins, it cannot produce histaminase, which protects the body from allergies.

When the digestive system is functioning properly and the colon is working every day, allergies will gradually disappear.

FOODS TO HEAL—Sprouts, almonds, beans, raw nuts, peas. Lemons, sesame seeds, green leafy vegetables, root vegetables, buckwheat, yellow fruits and vegetables. Berries, carrots, apricots, parsley, celery, cabbage, watercress, apples, grapes, onions, artichokes, garlic. Magnesium food prevents allergies: almonds, whole grains, cashews, sesame seed, lima, white,and red beans, millet, bananas, wild rice, brown rice. Sodium is found in zucchini, celery, carrots, beets and seaweeds.

VITAMINS AND MINERALS—Multi-vitamins with extra A, B-complex (pantothenic acid, B6, Bl2), Vitamin C with bioflavonoids, (helps in assimilation of iron). Multi-minerals with extra calcium and magnesium (balanced), (magnesium prevents allergies, manganese, potassium, zinc. Iodine (kelp), is necessary to produce thyroid hormone, to protect metabolism. Sodium (natural in herbs and food), prevent water getting into the cells, which results in stuffy nose, watery eyes and swollen tissues.

Pantothenic acid, vitamin C and vitamin E have all been shown to reduce the production of histamine under stress.

HERBAL COMBINATIONS—Allergy, Bone, Digestion, Lungs, Lower Bowel formulas. Herbal formulas will help clean and strengthen the mucus membranes.

SINGLE HERBS-Alfalfa (Acid/alkaline balance), burdock (with dandelion strengthen the liver), chaparral (cleans deep in the cells), chickweed, comfrey, dandelion, echinacea, eyebright, fenugreek (cleans the stomach of mucus), gentian (tonic for the intestinal tract), golden seal (antibiotic, congestion), gotu kola (feeds the brain), hops (sedative, headaches), ho-shou-wu, irish moss, lobelia, ma hueng (natural antihistamine), myrrh, parsley, psyllium, red raspberry, scullcap, slippery elm, wood betony, wormwood, yellow dock.

SUPPLEMENTS—Amino acids (histidine, isoleucine, tryptophan, tyrosine), Bee pollen acidophilus (milk-free), Bentonite, Fish Oil Lipids, Salmon Oil, Evening primrose oil (essential fatty acids are needed to produce adrenal hormones and to synthesize pantothenic acid in the intestines), Rice Bran Syrup, Royal Jelly, Glucomannan. Digestive enzymes (to aid in digestion to prevent toxins from accumulating in the blood).

AVOID—Any foods that provoke allergic symptoms; (introduce back into diet one at a time after one month of complete abstention from them). Common allergenic foods include: wheat products, corn products, chocolate, dairy products, white potatoes, tomatoes and tobacco (night shade family). Avoid MSG, nitrates, artificial food colors or flavors, chemically grown or sprayed foods (also grains), processed oils or refined flour. Strong spices overstimulates the adrenals. Stay away from sugar, coffee and alcohol.

ALZHEIMER'S DISEASE

This disease is characterized by progressive degeneration of the brain, memory and nervous system. Studies indicate that high aluminum concentrations in the brain tissue may be one causative factor. Another may be the diminished activity of the neurotransmitter acetylcholine. Neurotransmitters are chemicals located at the ends of brain nerve cells which make message transmission possible.

The brain is very susceptible to nutritional deficiencies and also to environmental toxins. The brain is sensitive to toxins created in an unhealthy colon. An unhealthy bloodstream can carry toxins to the brain and nervous system and cause brain cells to die.

This is a devastating disease that affects the families of the victims. It brings heartache, discomfort, frustration and hopelessness to those involved. New light and beliefs are being shed on diseases affecting the nervous system and brain. Many of these disorders can be prevented, delayed or controlled with nutritional supplements. The brain suffers when nutrients are lacking, especially the essential minerals.

NATURAL THERAPY—Oral Chelation, using vitamins, minerals, herbs, amino acids have been successful in cleaning the veins. Choline, found in lecithin, stimulates production of acetylcholine and improves Alzheimer's victims short term memory. Cleansing the liver and the bowels is beneficial. Low fat diet and exercise is helpful.

FOODS TO HEAL—A high fiber diet is important. Fresh fruits and vegetables, green leafy vegetable salads, using different kinds of cabbage (red, green, chinese), broccoli, asparagus, carrots, cauliflower, sprouts, seeds, nuts, cold pressed oils, lemons, oranges, grapefruit. Millet, buckwheat, brown rice, a lot of lightly steamed vegetables, fish. Sulphur foods acts as chelating agents: Watercress, brussels sprouts, horseradish, cabbage, turnip, cauliflower, raspberry, spinach, kelp, parsnip, leeks, garlic, onions, chives, swiss chard, okra. Distilled water has a chelating effect on the veins.

VITAMINS AND MINERALS—B-complex vitamins (with extra thiamine, B6, niacin, B15). Vitamin C, calcium and magnesium may help reduce accumulated aluminum as well as prevent it from accumulating.

Vitamin E helps transport oxygen to the brain cells. Vitamin E may also lower possibility of onset of Alzheimer's.

Minerals are essential for a healthy nervous system and brain. Copper, manganese, magnesium, iodine, silver and zinc play a vital role in memory and brain function. These are some of the elements that are in some way interdependent, and it's not possible to determine which one is the most important. Selenium, iodine and potassium are important for continued brain function. Minerals improve overall health of the body.

Sulphur is found and needed mostly in the nervous system and brain. It purifies and activates the body. Phosphorus nourishes the brain and nerves and stimulates the thinking process.

HERBAL COMBINATIONS—Liver, Lower Bowels, Immune, Nerves, Potassium. Stress and Anti-Plague formulas containing garlic help protect the immune system, which is also part of the nervous system and the brain.

SINGLE HERBS—Alfalfa, Burdock, Butcher's Broom (improves circulation), Capsicum (supplies nutrients to the brain), Chaparral (cleans heavy metals form the blood), Echinacea, Garlic (dissolves cholesterol and loosens it out of the arteries), Ginger, Ginseng (increases brain efficiency, improves concentration), Ginkgo (strengthen brain function), Gotu Kola (feeds the brain), Ho Shou-Wu, Lady's Slipper (feeds the nervous system), Passion Flower, Prickly Ash (increases circulation, cleans veins), Psyllium (helps clean the pockets in the colon of toxins), Rosemary, Red Clover, Scullcap, Suma (increases brain function), Valerian, Wood Betony.

SUPPLEMENTS—Co Q10 (carries oxygen to brain), Germanium (oxygen), Lecithin, RNA nutrients (sardines, spirulina, chlorella and bee pollen), Free form amino acids, Salmon Oil, Blue-green Algae.

AVOID—All aluminum products. Aluminum is found in most baking powders, cheese sauces, pickles, many salad dressings, table salt, white flour, fruit juices stored in aluminum cans, water from most municipal sources. It is found in some medicines. It is found in aspirin, antiperspirants, douches and feminine hygiene products, lipstick, antidiarrheal medications, and antacids. It is also found in many other products.

Avoid all foods that lower the immune system: sugar, white flour products,alcohol, tobacco, caffeine, additives and preservatives. Avoid red meat, its by-product is uric acid, and it is very hard to digest. If you use meat, obtain organic grown without antibiotics and hormones. Avoid all processed food the body needs essential nutrients for a healthy brain and nervous system.

ANEMIA

Symptoms of anemia include fatigue, loss of appetite, irritability, general weakness, pale skin and fingernails and headaches. Lack of or poor assimilation of B-12 or iron can cause anemia. Healthy blood is the life-line to all the organs of the body. An imbalanced diet, poor digestion and wrong food combining adds up to poor blood and anemia.

Anemia can also occur from recurrent infections or diseases involving the entire body. It also can happen with excessive losses of blood through such conditions as heavy menstruation or peptic ulcers.

NATURAL THERAPY—Blood Purifiers. The blood transports nutrients, hormones, electrolytes and waste material to and from every cell in the body; an imbalance or lack of nutrients leads to many problems and symptoms. Herbal therapies to tone up the glands, the circulatory system and the digestive tract.

FOODS TO HEAL—Whole grains, blackberries, cherries, blackstrap molasses, dried apricots (rich in iron), peaches, raisins, prunes, sunflower seeds, sesame seeds, egg yolks, fish, sprouts, beets, millet, buckwheat, yams, sweet potatoes, squash, plums, potatoes (with skins), red cabbage.

Enjoy all natural food, using a variety of fresh fruit, vegetables and sprouts. Fresh green salads will nourish and feed the blood.

VITAMINS AND MINERALS—Iron, protein, copper, folic acid and vitamins B6, B12, and C are all essential for the formation of red blood cells. Vitamin E may be needed to help maintain the health of the red blood cells. Vitamin A, B-Complex (extra B6, B12, PABA and pantothenic acid), C (with bioflavonoids-aids in assimilation of iron). E (carries oxygen to the cells). Calcium and magnesium (balanced), copper iron and zinc.

HERBAL COMBINATIONS-Anemia, Blood Purifier, Digestion and Liver.

SINGLE HERBS—Key herbs: Yellow Dock (40 percent iron) and Dandelion (help the liver assimilate iron), Alfalfa, Kelp, Dong Quai and Watercress. Barberry, Black Walnut, Burdock, Cayenne, Chaparral, Echinacea, Garlic, Gentian (helps in digestion), Ginger, Golden Seal, Hawthorn, Lobelia, Red Clover, Sarsaparilla.

SUPPLEMENTS—Beet powder (nourishes the blood), Chlorophyll, Blackstrap Molasses, Spirulina, Evening Primrose Oil, Blue-green algae.

AVOID—Coffee, black or green tea, white flour products, fried foods, excess fats and starches, excess protein, refined sugar, preservatives food and additives, canned foods, pasteurized milk.

ANOREXIA NERVOSA
(Bulimia)

Anorexia Nervosa and Bulimia are eating disorders. Anorexia is a disorder mainly with young girls who starve themselves for thinness. One-third of those involved die. It seems to be more than a desire for thinness; some feel that it is a way to return to their younger years where they didn't have to grow up.

Bulimia is characterized by binge-eating, then vomiting or using cathartics or diuretics. This involves those who feel emotional stress, frustration, low self-esteem, loneliness, depression, emptiness, and perfectionism. This disease of striving to lose weight may be a way to gain approval and elevate self-esteem.

Starvation and purging is a very dangerous practice that will bring long-lasting health problems or even coma and death. Vomiting often leads to deterioration of the stomach and esophagus linings, an increase in cavities and gum disease and even the loss of teeth. It flushes essential minerals from the body which are necessary for proper metabolism and physical and mental well-being.

Extreme restriction on calorie intake can cause fluid and electrolyte disturbances leading to heart problems, kidney failure and urinary infections. It can lead to any auto-immune disease as well as lower the immune system for germs and viruses to take over.

The brain is also disturbed and can cause shrinkage of the brain mass in eating disorder victims. The body begins to cannibalize itself when it has no other source of nourishment. Muscle mass is depleted and the heart muscle can atrophy.

NATURAL THERAPY—Herbs to improve digestion, the nervous system and the glandular system. Education on the importance of good nutrition has to be stressed. How the lack of minerals, especially zinc and potassium can put a strain on the heart as well as other organs. The lack of copper, depleted through vomiting is one example of how a small amount is essential to the body and when lacking causes many body dysfunctions. All minerals are essential and when depleted from the body causes destruction of the cells and organs.

FOODS TO HEAL—Foods high in copper are leeks, garlic, artichoke, parsley, beet root, dandelion greens and broccoli. The following foods are high in minerals: almonds, whole grains, molasses, egg yolks, green leafy vegetables, apricots and black figs.

VITAMINS AND MINERALS—Multi-vitamin and mineral supplement. A, B-complex, C (with bioflavonoids, D, and E. Calcium and magnesium (balanced), potassium, sodium, zinc (which is quickly lost during starvation).

HERBAL COMBINATIONS—Digestion, Glands, Hypoglycemia, and Nerves. Stress and Immune formulas will fortify the system.

SINGLE HERBS—Alfalfa (very rich in minerals), Black Cohosh (protects the female organs), Black Walnut (help balance minerals), Burdock (purifies the blood), Catnip (relaxes the nerves), Chamomile (rich in calcium and relaxing for the nerves), Chaparral, Dandelion (feed and protects the liver), Echinacea, Ginger (calms the stomach and helps in digestion), Ginseng (strengthens the whole body), Gotu Kola (feeds the brain), Hops (rebuilds the nerves), Ho Shou-Wu, Kelp, Lady's Slipper (healing for the brain), Licorice (provides energy and balances hormones), Lobelia, Papaya, Passion Flower, Peppermint, Scullcap (rebuild and nourish the nerves), Red Clover, Wild Yam, Wood Betony, Yellow Dock.

SUPPLEMENTS-These are vital when the body has been stripped and depleted of essential nutrients: Free-form amino acids, Evening Primrose, Oil, Fish Oil Lipids, Acidophilus, Green Drinks, Salmon Oil. Germanium, CO Q10 to supply oxygen to the cells. Blue-green Algae will build up the immune system. Liquid Chlorophyll will help build and purify the blood. A liquid mineral and herbal formula will help restore mineral imbalance.

AVOID—All processed food, it is essential to eat live food high in vitamins and minerals. Avoid caffeine, alcohol, tobacco, white sugar products: they all deplete more minerals from the body. Avoid meat which is high in uric acid and fat.

APPENDICITIS

Appendicitis is a disease of constipation and incomplete elimination. It is an autointoxication, a self poisoning from poor elimination. The appendix is needed in the body to help clean the cells so the lymphatic system can do its job of in the body to help clean the cells so the lymphatic system can do its job of filtering the toxins.Appendicitis is inflammation of the vermiform appendix due to an obstruction. It can occur at any age. It is responsible for the most common major surgical disease. If the appendix ruptures or perforates, the infected contents spill into the abdominal cavity, causing peritonitis, which is a very dangerous complication of appendicitis.

The appendix is lymph tissue and the lymphatic system helps protect the body from infections. If the appendix is removed the natural immune system is impaired. The appendix and tonsils become inflamed from lymphatic system congestion. When toxins are eliminated from the lymphatic system the inflammation of the appendix and tonsils usually clear up. Removing the appendix or the tonsils interfere with the body's ability to respond in a natural way to temporary toxic congestion.

NATURAL THERAPY—Cleaning the bowels and the blood and the liver. A pure water fast with psyllium to increase bulk. Potassium broths made with onions, celery, potatoes (peels), parsley. A fast using fresh lemons, pure maple syrup and cayenne pepper in pure water is cleansing and healing to the body.

FOODS TO HEAL—A high fiber diet to increase bulk and prevent retention and incomplete elimination of the bowels. High fiber foods are whole grains (barley, buckwheat, millet, whole wheat, cornmeal), brown rice, beans and lentils, vegetables such as cabbage, asparagus, carrots, green peas, spinach, onions, potatoes. Berries have a high content of fiber.

Use fresh green salads daily, using leaf lettuce, cabbage, carrots, broccoli and any fresh vegetables.

VITAMINS AND MINERALS—Vitamin A and C to fight infection. Minerals selenium and zinc for healing. A multi-vitamin and mineral supplement.

HERBAL COMBINATIONS—Infection fighters, Immune, Nervous, Liver and Lower Bowels.

SINGLE HERBS—Aloe Vera (acts as a laxative and is healing), Burdock (blood cleanser), Cayenne, Chaparral (cleans deep in the cells), Comfrey (healing for the mucus membranes), Echinacea (clean the lymphatics), Garlic, Golden Seal (will clean and purify the blood), Kelp (supplies minerals for healing), Myrrh, Pau D'Arco (cleans the blood and protects the liver), Rose Hips, Slippery Elm (healing and nourishing), Yellow Dock (rich in iron).

SUPPLEMENTS—Aloe Vera Juice (internally), Acidophilus, Chlorophyll (to clean the blood), Lecithin, Blue-green algae.

AVOID—Too much meat, potatoes and gravy diet. Low fiber food.

Stay away from sugar and white flour products, as well as deep fried food, (fried oils cannot metabolize in the body).

ARTERIOSCLEROSIS
(Hardening of the arteries)

Plaques and deposits of fatty elements on blood vessel walls contributes to this circulatory disorder. It can hinder the flow of blood, thus leading to high blood pressure, strokes and heart attacks. This is called the silent killer, because it is a slow build up on the artery walls. The accumulation usually starts around the heart first, then the arteries. It is known that fatty streaks are found in the aortas (main artery of the body) of children in almost every country and it is believed that the fatty streaks are the precursors of plaques. I believe this is caused from poor elimination and a dysfunctioning of the gall bladder and the liver.

The liver, under normal circumstances, can eliminate toxins from the body. But when the liver is overburdened with toxins from the bowels that have not completely eliminated it has to try to detoxify excess poisons. The liver has to dump the excess poisons into the bile. This thickens the bile and clogs the gall bladder. Since the liver is responsible for dealing with cholesterol, it cannot filter it properly when it is overloaded.

NATURAL THERAPY—Blood purification, cleaning the bowels and short fasts. Herbal therapies on the circulation, glands and muscular systems. Changing the diet to high fiber foods, fruits, and a lot of vegetables. Using nuts, seeds and sprouts to obtain protein.

FOODS TO HEAL—Garlic, onions, salmon, sardines, cod, (or consuming Omega 3 oil). Eat food containing nucleic acid: they build cell energy to help retard deterioration of the arteries. They help repair the DNA and RNA. They are: asparagus, beets, whole grains, chick peas, kidney beans, honey, lentils, lima beans, millet, buckwheat, nuts, sardines, salmon, split peas, soy beans, tuna, leafy vegetables.

VITAMINS AND MINERALS—Multi-vitamin, B-complex (extra B6 and niacin), Vitamin C (with bioflavonoids), E (increases oxygen), choline, inositol (help dissolve plaque, found in lecithin), Calcium (herbal) magnesium, chromium, selenium and zinc.

HERBAL COMBINATIONS—Blood Purifier, Bone Combination, Heart, Chelation, Lower Bowel formulas.

SINGLE HERBS—Alfalfa, Aloe Vera (cleansing affect on the veins), Black Walnut, Burdock, Capsicum (Equalizes blood circulation and cleans veins), Chaparral (cleans deep in tissues), Cascara Sagrada (prevent toxins from accumulating in blood and cholesterol adhering to walls of the veins), Comfrey (cleans up dead tissues), Echinacea, Garlic and Parsley (work together to prevent plaque build-up), Golden Seal, Hawthorn (strengthens heart and supplies oxygen to blood), Horsetail (supplies silicon, calcium and other minerals),

Juniper Berries, Irish Moss, Kelp, Licorice, Marshmallow, Pau D'Arco, Psyllium, Red Clover, Slipper Elm, Watercress, Yellow Dock.

SUPPLEMENTS—The amino acid alanine reduces cholesterol when combined with arginine and glycine. L-carnitine, cysteine, glutamine and methionine prevent accumulation of fat in the liver. Taurine, Lecithin, Evening Primrose, Oil, Salmon Oil, Co Q10, Fish Oil Lipids, Germanium (lowers cholesterol), Aloe Vera Juice. Digestive Enzymes are important for proper digestion.

AVOID—Red meat (too much, high in fat), white flour and sugar products, salt, high fat foods, animal fats and shortenings, fried foods, doughnuts, pastries, all deep-fat fried foods. Avoid alcohol, caffeine, soft drinks, tea, white sugar, white flour products. Avoid constipation, toxins can back-up into the blood- stream and cause other problems.

ARTHRITIS

(also bursitis, gout, rheumatism)

These disorders are characterized by inflammation of the joints. They can be caused by excessive calcium deposits, causing spurs or deposits of crystallized uric acids in the joints that irritate and cause pain. Research indicates that many arthritic conditions can be allergy-related. Elimination of certain dietary elements may prove very helpful. Arthritis is an accumulation of toxic waste in the body. It can accumulate over a period of years if the diet is too acid. We can inherit a weak body with the tendency to arthritis.

Rheumatoid arthritis is a chronic, inflammatory disorder causing stiffness, deformity and pain to joints and muscles. It is an auto-immune disease where the body attacks itself as if it is a threat to the body. It can affect the lungs, blood vessels, the spleen, skin and muscles. Early signs can be fatigue, muscular aches and pains, stiffness in the joints, and swelling.

Osteoarthritis is a wearing-away ailment. Cartilage in the joints wastes away; calcium spurs may form on surfaces which contact bones.

The symptoms of these diseases are a stagnation of blood, lymphatics, and the nervous system. Poor diet and stress can predispose one to them.

NATURAL THERAPY—Herbal therapy to treat the skeletal/muscular, circulation, glands, and the nervous system. A basic alkaline diet, the body becomes "acidic" and the cartilage in the joints begins to dissolve because of acid in the blood. Blood purification is indicated. Use cleansing diets, short juice fasts (carrot & celery), and cleanse the bowels. Distilled water acts as a chelating agent. Minerals are vital; the best kind are in herbs. An herbal liquid formula with minerals is excellent.

FOODS TO HEAL—Fresh vegetable juices, fresh fruits, whole grains, okra, sprouts, yogurt, blackstrap molasses, cherries (especially for gout). Red cherry juice (non sweetened) eliminates uric acid.

Whey powder, okra and celery are high in sodium to prevent and dissolve deposits in the joints. Bean sprouts, onions, cabbage, avocado, parsley, watercress, endive, yellow corn meal, barley, steamed brown and wild rice, millet. Winter squash, Green salads and potato peeling broth.

VITAMINS AND MINERALS—A, B-Complex (extra B6, B12, niacin, pantothenic acid). Vitamin E. Calcium and magnesium (herbal calcium formula), selenium, silicon, manganese and zinc.

HERBAL COMBINATIONS—Blood Purifier, Bone Combination, Comfrey Pepsin, Digestion, Nerve, Pain.

SINGLE HERBS—Key herbs-Alfalfa (helps ease pain, mineral content helps maintain acid/alkaline balance), Chaparral (cleans deep in the muscles and joints), Comfrey (helps build new tissue), Dandelion, Devil's Claw (reduces inflammation and heals), Hydrangea (contains cortisone like properties), Kelp (rich in minerals for healing), Yucca (stimulates natural cortisone), Aloe Vera, Brigham Tea, Burdock, Capsicum, Dulse, Garlic, Parsley, Papaya, Saffron (helps the body utilize oils), Red Clover, Watercress, White Willow (helps in pain).

SUPPLEMENTS—Free-form amino acids, Cystine (works with pantothenic acid in arthritis treatment). Histidine (removes heavy metals), Phenylalanine (for pain), Distilled water, Green Drinks, Juices (carrot and celery), Co Q10, Fish Oil Lipids, Salmon Oil, Evening Primrose Oil, Rice Bran Syrup, Chinese Essential oils and Tea Tree Oil (external), Lecithin (helps control the chemical balance of the joints).

AVOID—Red meat, white flour, white sugar, salt, cola drinks, fried foods, pork, fats, heated oils, citrus fruit, nightshade family foods (tobacco, tomatoes, potatoes, green peppers, eggplant), Dairy products, potato starch (in canned and packaged foods), environmental pollutants.

Avoid digestive disturbances; they lead to a loss of nutrients because of poor digestion and assimilation. Undigested food ferments in the intestinal tract and toxins can enter the blood stream.

ASTHMA

This is a chronic, usually allergic, condition which causes difficulty in breathing and wheezing, due to mucus and inflammation in the lungs. The body is congested with toxins and excess mucus. When the bowels are congested the lungs try to eliminate. The lungs shouldn't have to eliminate; they are sensitive and this is why they become irritated. Allergies are caused by the irritated mucous membranes. This is considered an emotional disease. Resolving emotions have a positive effect on asthma.

The lungs are one of the organs of elimination. Breathing properly is essential to cleanse the body of toxins, as well as help the body utilize nutrients. Exercising in fresh air helps the lungs increase their ability to pump oxygen. The vessels and circulation are kept healthy by the blood vessels.

Incomplete digestion, poor nutrition and autointoxication, along with free radicals and rancid fats, can result in particles of matter which gradually close the "pores". The lungs then lose their elasticity

Air pollution can cause and worsen respiratory illnesses, including asthma, bronchitis, and pneumonia. Fine particulate matter (toxins in the air), suppresses the body's immune system and may even cause cancer. Ozone is a very serious pollutant that can cause permanent lung scarring and decreased pulmonary function. Carbon monoxide binds with hemoglobin in the blood system. This decreases the ability of the blood to transport oxygen and can result in dizziness, headaches and slowed reflexes. Prolonged exposure to carbon monoxide may cause arterial or heart disease.

NATURAL THERAPY—Lower bowel cleansing would be the most beneficial. Read information on Autointoxication. Herbal therapy to clean and strengthen the lungs. Short fasts, cleansing diets and a positive attitude will speed the healing.

FOODS TO HEAL—Green leafy vegetables, sprouts, whey, yogurt, okra, sunflower seeds, black beans, onions, garlic, honey. Fresh fruits and vegetables, nuts, seeds, oatmeal (thermos cooking), brown rice and whole grains.

VITAMINS AND MINERALS—Vitamin A (50,000 units to heal), B-complex to strengthen the nervous system, (extra B6, necessary due to metabolism deficiency), B12, PABA (pantothenic acid), C (with bioflavonoids) helps combat stress, E (low doses at the beginning). Calcium (to rebuild and relax the nerves), and magnesium, manganese, herbal potassium (helps control mucus production), selenium, zinc.

HERBAL COMEINATIONS—Allergies, Digestion, Lungs, Nerves, Lower Bowels.

SINGLE HERBS—Key Herbs: Capsicum (dissolves mucus), Cascara Sagrada (keeps the bowels clean), Comfrey, Fenugreek (dissolves mucus, contains natural dehydrating properties, cleanses the kidneys), Garlic (clears congestion from the lungs), Horseradish (very healing for the lungs), Lobelia (calming and cleansing for the lung), Slippery Elm, Alfalfa, Aloe Vera (soothing and healing for the lungs), Bayberry, Black Cohosh, Ephedra (bronchial dilator and decongestant), Burdock, Chaparral, Chickweed, Dandelion, Echinacea, Eyebright, Ginseng, Golden Seal (expectorant, soothes inflamed mucous membranes, good for infections), Gotu Kola, Horsetail, Ho Shou-Wu, Licorice, Marshmallow (relaxes bronchial tubes removes hardened phlegm and soothes irritated tissues in the lungs), Ma Hueng, Mullein, Oat Straw, Pau D'Arco, Red Clover, Rose Hips, Scullcap, Valerian, White Willow, Wood Betony, Yarrow, Yellow Dock.

SUPPLEMENTS—Free-form Amino Acids to build new tissues: Glutathione, Histidine and Isoleucine to regulate glands. Chlorophyll, Lemon juice, RNA-DNA foods: Sardines, Spirulina, Bee Pollen, tincture of Lobelia for emergency, Evening Primrose Oil, Fish Oil Lipids, Salmon Oil.

AVOID—Salt, starches, milk, chocolate, eggs, sugar, white flour, red meats. MSG (monosodium glutamate). Sulfites, preservatives in processed foods, dried fruits and some restaurant salads. Food colorings are suspected to be a contributor to asthma.

ATHLETE'S FOOT

This is a fungus infection of the skin of the feet, mainly between the toes. It thrives in warm and damp pla es. It is commonly transmitted from person to person through towels and locker rooms or bathroom floors. This fungus spreads quickly when our friendly bacteria is destroyed by antibiotics, sugar diet, drugs, and radiation.

NATURAL THERAPY—Purify the blood and cleanse the colon. A balanced diet. Soaking the feet in water with antifungal herbs, such as Pau D'Arco Tea. Also drink the Pau D'Arco tea, about 6 cups daily.

FOODS TO HEAL—Pure water, fresh fruits and vegetables, whole grains, yogurt (unsweetened), garlic, lemon juice on the infected area. Tea Tree Oil on the feet is beneficial.

VITAMINS AND MINERALS—Vitamin A and C for healing the tissues and to stimulate the immune system. B-complex vitamins (yeast free), Minerals: Selenium (strengthens the immune system) and zinc (heals skin problems).

HERBAL COMBINATIONS—Blood Purifier, Candida Formulas, Cleansing, Immune, Nerve and Stress combinations.

SINGLE HERBS—Key Herbs: Black Walnut (extract to use externally, will kill fungus infections), Chaparral (antiseptic), Echinacea (natural antibiotic), Garlic (antibiotic), Pau D'Arco (blood cleanser), Red Clover. Alfalfa, Capsicum, Dandelion, Don Quai, Hops, Horsetail (contains silicon and calcium to heal skin problems), Kelp, Lady's Slipper, Licorice, Mistletoe, Passion Flower, Sarsaparilla, Scullcap, Valerian, White Oak (use externally, as antiseptic), Yellow Dock (rich in iron for healing).

SUPPLEMENTS—Acidophilus, Liquid Chlorophyll, Caprylic Acid, Salmon Oil, Evening Primrose Oil, Tea Tree Oil (external).

AVOID—Meat, sugar products of all kinds. Rich foods, salt, white flour products.

AUTISM

This is a type of mental illness which causes a person to withdraw into a private fantasy world, not being able to communicate with others in a real environment. Autistic people are not responsive to love and affection. Some of the children have low IQ's but some have normal ones.

NATURAL THERAPY—Blood purification, bowel cleaning, and brain and nervous system stimulation. Make sure natural foods are given to children with autism. Nutrition is very important. The B-complex vitamins with extra B6 and magnesium have produced good results. Keeping food colorings and preservatives from the diet.

FOODS TO HEAL—Fresh fruit and vegetables, sprouts, whole grains (cooked in thermos), brown rice, millet, buckwheat, whole oats.

VITAMINS AND MINERALS—Vitamin A builds the immune system, B-complex vitamins are essential for normal brain and nervous system function, extra B6 (deficiency has been linked to autism), vitamin C (with bioflavonoids), vitamin E improves brain function (aids circulation). All minerals are important for brain function.

Calcium needs hydrochloric acid for assimilation. It calms nerves.

Magnesium calms the nerves. Iron increases resistance to stress and disease. Selenium builds the immune system, retards formation of free radicals, and helps oxidation of cells. Silicon is essential for all connective tissue health. Zinc is needed in the brain and nervous system.

HERBAL COMBINATIONS—Blood Purification, Bowels, Circulation, and the Nerves.

SINGLE HERBS—Key Herbs: Gotu Kola (brain food), Ginkgo (increases circulation), Hawthorn, Capsicum, Lady's Slipper (good for brain function), Alfalfa, Black Walnut, Dandelion, Echinacea (blood cleanser), Garlic, Hops (nerves), Licorice, Lobelia, Red Clover, Scullcap (strengthens nerves), Wood Betony.

SUPPLEMENTS—Amino acid Glutamine improved I.Q. in some retarded children. Evening Primrose Oil, Salmon Oil, Spirulina, Bee Pollen, Rice Bran Syrup, Blue-green Algae.

AVOID—Check for heavy metal accumulation. Allergies can be involved in retardation. Avoid all processed food, sugar, white flour products, caffeine, soft drinks, candy, chocolate, cake, cookies, pastries.

BACKACHE
(Aches and Pains)

Pain is the way the body is telling you something is wrong. The brain tells you from the response triggered by the pain to be aware of a certain area in the body. Aches are not as serious as pain and there are many different levels of aches and pains. Lower back pain can originate from constipation. Chiropractic treatments along with nutritional knowledge have helped many people cure their aches and pains. Headaches can also be caused by constipation, and digestion problems can produce headaches. Stress can cause weakness in the body and create pain. Anger, frustration, grief, severe disappointment and anxiety can create pain in a weak spot in our body. People in poor health usually have aches and pains.

Are pain killers the answer? Americans spend millions of dollars each year on pain relievers. These pain pills usually give moderate relief with exposure to possible serious side effects.

Ibuprofen has been known to cause liver cells to die. There have been thousands of reported cases of liver damage caused by acetaminophen listed in scientific literature. Acetaminophen in the Physician's Desk Reference list over 100 drugs. This is a drug that relieves pain and reduces fever. Ibuprofen is one of the drugs listed under acetaminophen. This drug also can cause kidney damage and encourage the formation of scar tissue in kidney cells.

The best method in dealing with aches and pains is to prevent them through a healthier life style.

NATURAL THERAPY—Clean the lower bowels, purify the blood strengthen the nerves, bones and muscles. Chiropractor adjustments are very beneficial. Change diet to live foods.

FOODS TO HEAL—Whole grains (cooked in thermos to protect live enzymes), sprouts, fresh vegetables and fruit. Calcium foods: Sesame seeds, kelp, irish moss, dulse, collard leaves, kale, turnip greens, almonds, parsley, watercress, chickpeas, beans, sunflower seeds, okra, endive.

VITAMINS AND MINERALS—Vitamin C, iron and manganese are essential for production of new collagen (holds us together), Calcium is needed (herbal is better). Zinc is necessary to maintain all tissues. Protein assimilation is essential.

HERBAL COMBINATIONS—Bone, Digestion, Lower Bowels, Nerves, Pain.

SINGLE HERBS—Key Herbs: comfrey (builds new tissues), Horsetail, (contains calcium and minerals for healing) Oatstraw, Slippery Elm (rich in protein and healing properties). Alfalfa (rich in minerals), Aloe Vera, Burdock, Dandelion, Hops (relaxing), Lady's Slipper, Scullcap (strengthens the nerves, and helps pain, White willow (pain reliever).

SUPPLEMENTS—Herbal creams for pain (external), Chinese Essential Oils, Peppermint oil, Wintergreen oil.

AVOID—Heavy meat diet, constipation, drugs such as cortisone (destroy bones), bending forward without bending the knees. Also avoid lifting heavy objects. A heavy purse may injure the neck, shoulders and back.

BEDWETTING

Bedwetting can be a concern for parents, but they should be patient with the child. The child will be able to take the responsibility when he is old enough to understand. The child cannot help the bedwetting and should not be scolded or punished. Allergies have been implicated in bedwetting. It has been seen in children where there is a family history of allergies or hayfever.

Constipation can cause bedwetting (puts pressure on the bladder).

Bedwetting may be caused by er otional upsets, infections, or extreme tiredness (allergies can cause fatigue).

NATURAL THERAPY—Purifying the blood and strengthening the urinary tract. Using food and herbs to strengthen the bladder, kidneys and the nervous system.

FOODS TO HEAL—Foods high in calcium and magnesium. Magnesium foods: Kelp, almonds, cashews, soybeans (milk), dulse, sesame seeds, beans, millet, grains, wild rice. Calcium foods: sesame seeds, kelp, irish moss, dulse, collard greens, kale leaves, almonds, soybeans, parsley, watercress, sunflower seeds, broccoli.

VITAMINS AND MINERALS—Multi-Vitamin and Mineral supplement. Extra calcium and magnesium (herbal formula). Silicon, manganese and zinc will strengthen the bladder.

HERBAL COMBINATIONS—Bladder and kidneys, Bone combinations, Glands and Nerves.

SINGLE HERBS—Key herbs: Buchu (heal and strengthen the bladder), Cornsilk (cleans mucus membranes and heals), oatstraw (antiseptic properties), and Uva Ursi (cleans urinary tract). Other herbs that help: Dandelion, Hops, Marshmallow (soothing and healing), Parsley, (natural diuretic), Scullcap, Slippery Elm (healing and nourishing) and St. Johnswort.

SUPPLEMENTS—Bee Pollen, Evening Primrose Oil, Salmon Oil, Chlorophyll.

AVOID—Foods involved in allergies: Milk, chocolate, eggs, cereals, bread, corn, citrus fruits (unripened), food additives and colorings, carbonated and caffeine drinks. Avoid drinking before going to bed. Give nervine herbs during the day, at night the child may sleep too soundly.

BLADDER AND KIDNEY INFECTIONS

Cystitis is an inflammation of the bladder, and is usually caused by bacteria. Kidney infections can result and are more serious. Frequent urination, pain, burning discomfort and a dark-colored and scanty urine can be symptoms. Backache and fever can occur in young children, also vomiting, nausea and diarrhea. The main cause is toxemia with impure blood and too many sweet foods causing an overly acid condition.

The kidneys have the job of filtering waste products from the blood. The kidneys also regulate the fluid and electrolyte balance in the body. The bladder holds the urine and if toxins accumulate without being eliminated often, it can develop infections. Drinking plenty of pure water will help keep the bladder clean.

Autointoxication is one cause of bladder and kidney infections. Constipation causes a back-up in the bloodstream which irritates the bladder and causes irritations. Congested kidneys will cause the skin to try and eliminate. The skin is the largest elimination organ of the body and takes over if the kidneys are plugged up with mucous material and toxins.

The liver helps to detoxify and clean the blood and convert toxins into water soluble particles. The kidneys are the filters that collect toxic particles and pass them out of the body.

NATURAL THERAPY—Blood purification, Demulcent, Antibiotic and Antiseptic therapies. Juice fasting will help heal the kidneys and bladder. Liquid chlorophyll will purify the blood, pure apple juice, green drinks and citrus juices will cleanse and heal. Enemas or lower bowel cleansers in herbal formulas will also help eliminate toxins from the system.

FOODS TO HEAL—Garlic, onions, potassium broths (potato peelings, carrots tops, parsley, celery, etc.). Cherry and cranberry juices (unsweetened). Cranberry juice inhibits bacterial growth. Fresh lemon juice in pure water is healing.

VITAMINS AND MINERALS—Vitamin A, B-complex (extra B6, pantothenic acid, choline), Vitamin C with bioflavonoids and vitamin E, Calcium and magnesium (balance), manganese, potassium, selenium, zinc. Magnesium and vitamin D help to dissolve calcium deposits.

HERBAL COMBINATIONS—Bladder and Kidney, Digestion, Infections, Glands.

SINGLE HERBS—Key Herbs: Cornsilk (strengthens and heals), Garlic (natural antibiotic), Hydrangea (natural diuretic to clean the clogged up filter of the kidneys), Juniper Berries (natural diuretic, heals) Parsley (diuretic), and Uva Ursi (strengthens and tones the urinary system). Other herbs: Alfalfa, Burdock, Dandelion, Golden Seal (cleans and heals the urinary tract), Kelp, Marshmallow (soothing and healing), Pau D'Arco (cleans the blood), Red Raspberry, Rose Hips (rich in vitamin C for healing), Yarrow.

SUPPLEMENTS—Liquid Chlorophyll, Acidophilus, Flaxseed Tea, Amino Acids: L-Cysteine, and L-Methionine.

AVOID—Carbonated beverages, tea, coffee, alcohol and caffeine soft drinks. Avoid sugar products, it encourages infections. Avoid underwear which prevents air circulation (cotton is best). Toilet tissue should be used from the front to the back to prevent irritations and infections. Avoid constipation, this can cause irritations from a toxic build-up in the blood. Avoid a high milk diet, it is very rich in protein which will produce acid condition.

Avoid aspirin, researchers at the Oregon Health Sciences University in Portland said there is no doubt that aspirin, taken over a long period of time in a cumulative dose of more than two kilograms, can cause permanent kidney damage requiring dialysis or transplants. Three tablets a day for three years could yield harmful dosages.

BLOOD POISONING

(Gangrene, Tetanus)

Blood poisoning causes the blood to become infected and congested. This contamination can be carried to any part of the body. This occurs when the blood is over acid and congested with toxins. It is considered toxemia of the blood. When a red streak appears, it can be very serious and a natural health practitioner should be consulted.

Autointoxication is one cause of impure blood. This is a self-poisoning by way of the large colon. When constipation or incomplete elimination is present this cause a back-up into the bloodstream. This can happen even if you have three bowel movements a day if the colon doesn't completely eliminate. This is caused by eating junk food. White flour products, pasta, spaghetti, macaroni, cheese, dairy products will all cause constipation.

NATURAL THERAPY—Blood Purification. Teas using Echinacea, Pau D'Arco, or Red Clover Blend will enter the blood stream and clean and purify the blood. A juice fast will clean as well as build up the blood. Citrus juices will clean the toxins: orange, grapefruit, lemons and limes. External: Plantain poultice, clay packs and Black Walnut, Slippery Elm, moistened with Aloe Vera juice or pure water.

FOODS TO HEAL—Beets and beet greens, Swiss chard, alfalfa sprouts, parsley, cherries, grapes. Green drinks will help clean the blood. Blackstrap molasses is rich in iron and copper.

VITAMINS AND MINERALS—Vitamin A (100,00 units for a while), Vitamin C, every hour (watch for diarrhea, tolerance level) B-complex vitamins are involved with healing, especially B12 and folic acid (essential for the formation of healthy blood cells in the bone marrow). Selenium and zinc are healing. Vitamin C and E aids in the assimilation of organic iron. Iron obtained from Yellow Dock is natural. Copper transports nutrient-bearing oxygen to all parts of the body.

HERBAL COMBINATIONS—Blood Purifier, Bone Combination, Immune formula, Liver and Gallbladder, Lower Bowel.

SINGLE HERBS—Key Herbs: Burdock (one of the greatest blood cleansers), Chaparral (cleans blood and cells), Echinacea (lymphatic and blood cleanser), Garlic (cleans and purifies the blood), Golden Seal (cleans and purifies the digestive tract), Pau D'Arco (liver and blood purifier) drink it in tea form, Yellow Dock (rich in organic iron). Other important herbs: Alfalfa (rich in minerals), Bayberry, Black Walnut (kills parasites and worms), Butcher's Broom, Cascara Sagrada (keeps the bowels regular), Dandelion (liver cleanser), Fenugreek (loosens hard mucous), Kelp (cleans and nourishes the blood), Licorice, Sarsaparilla, Yarrow.

SUPPLEMENTS: Blue-green algae, Liquid Chlorophyll, Barley Juice, Lecithin. Hydrochloric Acid (insufficient will prevent the absorption of iron), Wheat grass juice.

AVOID—Junk food diet contributes to toxic blood. Avoid constipation. Avoid a low fiber diet. Avoid alcohol, drugs, vaccination (contains toxins and viruses), all sugar products (leaches nutrients from the body). High fat and meat diet will contribute to toxic blood.

BRONCHITIS

Bronchitis is a general term used to describe inflammation of the mucous membranes inside the bronchial tubes. The lubricating glands of the bronchi become enlarged, and the tiny hairs become clogged with mucus is cleared by coughing. The air chambers can become strained and weakened. Coughing can linger as long as three months after an acute attack of bronchitis.

It can be caused by polluted air or smoking which weakens the lungs. Allergies are often associated with bronchitis, however when the body is strengthened and the mucous membranes cleaned of toxins, both allergies and bronchitis will clear up. Constipation or incomplete elimination of the bowels are also connected with bronchitis. The lungs are one of the organs of elimination and when the colon is congested it can back-up into the lungs.

NATURAL THERAPY—Juice fasting along with enemas or bowel cleanser. The body becomes toxic, from too many acid foods. An alkaline diet after cleansing the body will build up the lungs. Exercise to build up the lungs, using deep breathing, will help protect from infections.

FOODS TO HEAL—Correct food combining will help heal the lungs. Incomplete digestion and poor nutrition can irritate the lungs. Citrus juices (tree ripened if possible)—Frozen juices are second best, if fruits are picked ripe and frozen. More alkaline foods, fresh and raw fruits and vegetables. Salads using several kinds of leafy lettuce and vegetables. Barley water with lemon juice, contains hordenine which relieves bronchial spasms. Cranberry juice (unsweetened) acts as an antiseptic.

VITAMINS AND MINERALS—Vitamin A (up to 100,000 I.U.), fish liver oils and beta carotene), B-complex (speeds healing), Vitamin C(with bioflavonoids, large amounts to start), D and E will also heal. Multi-mineral, extra iron (Yellow Dock and Dandelion), manganese, silicon, sodium, zinc.

HERBAL COMBINATIONS—Allergy, Blood Cleansers, Digestion, Lower Bowels, Lungs, Nerves.

SINGLE HERBS—Key Herbs: Boneset (helps aches), Cascara Sagrada, Comfrey, Garlic (antiseptic), Ginger, Lobelia (Chest constrictor), Marshmallow (soothing and healing), Mullein (heals lungs), Slippery Elm (supplies protein and heals). Also the following: Capsicum, Echinacea, Golden Seal, Eucalyptus, Licorice, Ma Hueng, Pau D'Arco.

SUPPLEMENTS—Hot Lemon Juice with Ginger, Liquid Chlorophyll, Royal Jelly, Bee Propolis, Blue-green algae.

AVOID—Too much intake of starchy foods, salt, sugar and meat. Cheese, fried foods, chocolate, pastries, refined cereals and pastas.

BRUISING

Bruising is bleeding under the skin. The underlying tissues are injured, which results in swelling, black and blue marks and pain. Increased bruising may be a result of anemia, malnutrition, overweight, and/or lack of vitamins and minerals. Too many drugs, such as aspirin can cause bruising.

NATURAL THERAPY—Blood building therapy and cleansing diet will help bruising. Eliminating acid forming foods and adding more alkaline foods to the diet. Cleansing the blood is important, for bruising can be a warning sign of cancer.

FOODS TO HEAL—Carrots, apricots, kale, spinach, collard greens, Swiss chard, beet greens, sprouts, wheat grass juice, grains (thermos cooking), chives, onions and garlic. Sesame Seeds (contain vitamin T, which helps build healthy blood platelets).

VITAMINS AND MINERALS—Vitamin A, C (with bioflavonoids), and vitamin K. Minerals: Multi -mineral, selenium, zinc.

HERBAL COMBINATIONS—Blood Cleanser, Bone, Digestion.

SINGLE HERBS—Key Herbs: Alfalfa, Horsetail (strengthens bones, flesh and cartilage), Kelp (healing and nourishing), Rose Hips (contains vitamin C and B-complex), Slippery Elm (heals skin), Yellow Dock (rich in iron and minerals). Other herbs to help: Black Walnut, Capsicum, Dandelion, Dong Quai (blood builder), Ginger, Hawthorn, Hops, Lady's Slipper, Lobelia, Marshmallow, Scullcap, St. Johnswort, White Oak Bark (heals skin).

SUPPLEMENTS—Liquid Chlorophyll; poultice of Comfrey and Black Walnut mixed with Aloe Vera Juice or pure water. Essential fatty acids. Redmond Clay externally. Blue-green algae.

AVOID—Smoking (depletes vitamin C), Drugs (some deplete nutrients). Aspirin, refined foods, caffeine (depletes minerals from the body). Anticlotting drugs can cause vessel rupture, clotting and thrombosis.

BURNS

Burns can cause damage to the tissues from heat, hot water, electricity, chemicals (acid or alkaline), or radiation. They can range from a mild burn to charring with destruction of the skin.

There are three basic types of burns. First degree which cause redness and some pain, second degree which cause redness and blisters, and third degree which cause destruction of the skin and underlying muscles.

The first positive action in treating burns is to apply cold water (Not ice water). Injury to the skin can be prevented if cold water is applied immediately.

NATURAL THERAPY—First, treat with cold water (apply cold water until pain has stopped). If it is from an acid or chemical, flush with water under the faucet to remove the irritating substance. First degree burns can be treated with Comfrey salves, Aloe Vera and Vitamin E. Second degree burns can be treated with a paste made from Comfrey, honey and wheat germ oil. Vitamin E can be used when it heals to prevent scarring. Third degree burns can be treated with the Comfrey paste, with honey and wheat germ oil. It is beneficial to have a live Aloe Vera plant and use it for emergencies.

FOODS TO HEAL—Almost all fresh green vegetables, freshly ground whole grains, cold pressed vegetable oils, bananas, green peas, oats, corn, raw fruits, sweet potatoes, egg yolks. Extra protein is needed, (soy protein drinks), and also a lot of liquids (pure water).

VITAMINS AND MINERALS— Vitamin A (100,000 I.U. daily for a while), Vitamin C (with bioflavonoids), very healing, B-complex (extra B12), E (used internally and externally). Multi-mineral supplement (burns heal faster when minerals are present), calcium and magnesium (balance), potassium, sodium, selenium, copper, zinc.

HERBAL COMBINATIONS—Bone (increases healing), Infections, Nerve and Relaxant combinations. Lower Bowel cleansers will help prevent infections.

SINGLE HERBS—Aloe Vera (very healing), Chickweed (will purify the blood), Comfrey (heal and restore damaged tissues), Garlic, Horsetail (contains silicon), Marshmallow (acid or fire burns), Oatstraw, Red Clover, Slippery Elm (internal and external). Witch Hazel, Yarrow.

SUPPLEMENTS—Aloe Vera Juice (decreases bacterial infections and speeds healing), Evening Primrose, Salmon Oil, Chinese essential oils (externally), Redmond Clay (make a paste), Tea Tree Oil (external).

AVOID—High sugar diet, sweet drinks, cortisone creams, ice water, acid foods (accumulates too many toxins in the body. Don't use butter or margarine, will cause burn to penetrate deeper.

CANCER

There are many different types of cancer. Some spread quickly and others take years to develop. The bloodstream and lymphatic system can take cancer cells to different parts of the body. Cancer is a severe disorder of the immune system, where the replication processes of the cells go haywire and reproduce wildly and invade other organs and tissues. This is known as malignancy.

The basic cause of cancer are those environmental, dietary and stress factors that allow normal cells to get out of control. Cancer is a risk all of us take because we cannot be at a well level all the time. Air pollution, pesticides, food additives and drugs, all contribute to the degree of health we can be at any one time.

NATURAL THERAPY—Blood purification and Nervine therapy, also the Lower Bowels and Liver should be the main concern. The nervine herbs will help strengthen the nervous system, which is connected to the immune system. The nerves help one cope with everyday stresses. When your nerves are strong and healthy the body can handle diet changes. The National Academy of Sciences validated what many nutritionally-oriented physicians have been saying for years: there is a connection between diet and cancer. The United States government has found evidence that there is a strong connection between diet and health, and now the American Cancer Society says that diet is a major cause of cancer. We can no longer deny the link between diet and cancer.

FOODS TO HEAL—A change of diet is necessary. Crucifers protect against cancer (cabbage, broccoli, brussels sprouts, cauliflower), because they encourage the formation of indole in our intestine which can help prevent colon cancer and some other cancers. High fiber diet will also protect against cancer. Foods rich in potassium: beans (sprout first), whole grains(best sprouted), wheat grass juice, almonds, sunflower and sesame seeds, lentils, parsley, blueberries, coconut, endive, leaf lettuce, oats (thermos cooking), potatoes (baked with skin), carrots, peaches, fresh fruits and vegetables. Buckwheat, brown rice and millet (easy to digest and assimilate).

VITAMINS AND MINERALS—Vitamin A (protects against bladder cancer), B-complex vitamins (fortifies the nerves), C (with bioflavonoids) (protects against all cancers), antioxidant, destroys, neutralizes and protects against additives, detoxify viruses and carcinogens which cause cancer, D, helps the body to use calcium, vitamin A and minerals. E, free radical scavenger (works with selenium), Multi-mineral, with extra calcium, magnesium, magnesium, selenium, silicon, zinc.

HERBAL COMBINATIONS—Blood Purifier, Bone, Candida, Cleansing, Digestion, General Cleanser, Glands, Immune, Lower Bowels, Nerves.

SINGLE HERBS—Key Herbs: Burdock (blood cleanser), Garlic (natural antibiotic), Capsicum (cleans the blood), Chaparral (cleans the blood and eliminates toxins), Echinacea (blood cleanser), Kelp (cleans and nourishes the blood), Lady's Slipper, Pau D'Arco (protects the liver and cleans the blood), Red Clover (cleans the blood), Suma (strengthens the whole body.

SUPPLEMENTS—Acidophilus, Liquid Chlorophyll, Blue-green algae.

Salmon oil and Evening Primrose Oil, Herbal teas containing Red Clover and Chaparral. Pau D'Arco Tea.

AVOID—Refined grains and sugars. Fried foods, and additives. Food colorings, coffee, tea, cola drinks. Avoid meat which is dead matter, cutting fats, and eliminating salt-cured, salt-pickled and smoked foods such as sausage, bacon, ham, smoked fish, bologna and hot dogs. Fluoride in water and toothpaste is linked to bone cancer. Breathing unhealthy air causes cancer, the toxins in the air are called "particulate matter". Obesity increases risk of colon cancer.

Smoking causes lung and mouth cancer. A high fat and meat diet can cause colon cancer.

CANDIDA
(also Thrush)

The overgrowth of the fungus Candida Albicans is known as Candidiasis. It debilitates the immune system. To get Candida under control, a person must adhere to a strict dietary regime.

Candida is a yeast infestation, called a parasite, which thrives in warm-blooded animals. (Scientifically classified as a fungus.) This fungus can cause thrush and vaginal infections, as well as spread to any part of the body that is weakened.

Candida multiplies and develops toxins which circulate in the bloodstream and cause all kinds of symptoms, and illness. It causes chemical reactions in the body. It can produce false estrogen and make the body think it has enough and signal the body to cease production. It also sends out messages to the thyroid making it think it has enough and therefore stopping thyroxin production. These results can cause menstrual irregularities and hypothyroid problems (see pamphlet, Candida Albicans: A Nutritional Approach by Louise Tenney).

NATURAL THERAPY—Cleansing the blood, the lower bowels, and improving digestion and liver function. Antibiotics is the main cause, destroying the friendly bacteria. Patience with diet will pay off in the long run.

FOODS TO HEAL—A change of diet to natural food. All vegetables, such as asparagus, broccoli, cabbage, greens of all kinds, cucumbers, peppers, lettuce, okra, beans, turnips, rutabagas, squash and potatoes. Onions, garlic, brussels sprouts, kohlrabi. Millet, brown rice, buckwheat, quinoa, amaranth. Unrefined oils such as safflower, soy, and olive oil. Wild rice dishes. Soak grains overnight before cooking or cook in thermos. Use millet or rice cakes instead of bread. Muffins also instead of bread. Sprouts. Fiber is important for cleansing the intestinal tract as well as absorb toxins.

VITAMINS AND MINERALS—Multi-vitamin and Mineral, natural and chelated, provides easier absorption. Vitamin A, heals, B-complex strengthens the nerves, high potency and yeast free. Vitamin C, flushes the cells, heals. Calcium and Magnesium balance, take with vitamin C, kelp and hydrochloric acid for better assimilation, Vitamin E increases body's resistance to stress and disease.

HERBAL COMBINATIONS—Blood Purifier, Candida Combination (with caprylic acid), Cleansing (cleans cells), Immune, Nervine, Stress.

SINGLE HERBS—Key Herbs: Black Walnut (kills parasites and fungus), Burdock (purifies blood), Chaparral (cleans deep in tissues), Dong Quai (blood purifier), Echinacea (cleans lymphatics and blood), Garlic (antibiotic), Licorice, Pau D'Arco (kills fungus), Red Clover (purifies the blood), White Oak. Other herbs: Alfalfa, Capsicum, Dandelion, Hops, Horsetail, Kelp, Mistletoe, Passion Flower, Sarsaparilla, Scullcap, Valerian, Yellow Dock.

SUPPLEMENTS—Acidophilus, Evening Primrose Oil, Salmon Oil, Caprylic Acid, Psyllium Hulls.

AVOID—Antibiotic therapy, Birth control pills, Cortisone, Progesterone suppositories, altered acid/alkaline balance, Meat, high mercury levels, aspirin, chlorine in water, chocolate, fluoride, sleeping pills, nitrates/nitrites, stress.

CARDIOVASCULAR DISORDERS

Heart disease, stroke and related disorders kill more Americans than all other causes of death combined. Heart attacks will strike and kill over 60,000 Americans this year. The heart accumulates fatty material around it before it accumulates on the veins; therefore it is usually advanced before you know you have heart trouble. Preventive measures can be taken before the heart is in serious trouble. One of the main causes, in my opinion is constipation. The bowels back up and the liver cannot eliminate fatty material and it accumulates in the blood and on the arteries.

NATURAL THERAPY—Blood purification, bowel cleansing and liver stimulation. Natural foods using a high fiber diet. Exercise will strengthen the lungs and heart.

FOODS TO HEAL—Whole grains(high in fiber). Cook in thermos overnight, (contains enzymes and B vitamins), brown rice, raw fruit and vegetables, sprouts (live enzymes), asparagus, apples, bananas, beans, buckwheat (strengthens veins), seeds and nuts, whey powder, yogurt.

VITAMINS AND MINERALS—A, B-complex (extra B3, B6, Bl2, pangamic acid, E (increases oxygen in blood), C (with bioflavonoids) cleans and strengthens the veins. Calcium and magnesium, copper, chromium, potassium, selenium (protects the heart), zinc.

HERBAL COMBINATIONS—Blood Purifier, Chelation, Digestion, Heart, Lower Bowel, Potassium.

SINGLE HERBS—Key Herbs: Hawthorn (feeds and protects the heart), Capsicum (cleans and nourishes the veins), Garlic (protects the veins), Burdock (blood cleanser), Butcher's Broom (strengthens the veins), Ginseng (protects the body), Gotu Kola (food for the brain, Horsetail, Mistletoe, Parsley, Saffron (helps digest oils). Other herbs: Black cohosh, Lobelia, Bugleweed, Blessed Thistle, Cramp Bark, Dandelion, Ephedra, Hops, Kelp, Lily of the Valley, Oatstraw, Passion Flower, Rose Hips, Scullcap, St. John's Wort, Valerian, Wood Betony, Yarrow.

SUPPLEMENTS—Chlorophyll, Lecithin, Flaxseeds, Evening Primrose Oil, Fish Oil Lipids, Salmon Oil, Blue-green Algae, Co Q10, Germanium, Glucomannan.

AVOID—Smoking, high meat diet, sugar (too much), constipation, liver congestion, caffeine, drugs, obesity, a sedentary lifestyle.

CARPAL TUNNEL SYNDROME

Carpal Tunnel Syndrome is a condition that occurs when the median nerve that runs through the carpal tunnel opening in the wrist gets pinched or pressured due to constant repetitive motions. It is seen in workers who perform repetitive tasks, such as painters, carpenters, typesetters, meat cutters, assembly-line workers, musicians, or computer workers.

The symptoms seem to be most severe at night. The pain will become so severe that it will awaken the sufferer. Symptoms include pain, numbness, tingling, and weakness in the hand muscles.

This disease is becoming more common with the computer age here to stay. Dr. Arnold Fox believes a low-fat diet will help. He has seen patients respond to diet change. Fatty deposits in the wrist seems to be the main cause. Prevention is more important than treating this syndrome.

NATURAL THERAPY—Blood Purification Therapy, Liver, and Lower Bowel Cleanser. Chelation Therapy has also helped many people.

FOODS TO HEAL—Brown rice, whole grains, soybeans, lentils, sunflower seeds, salmon, tuna, avocados, beans, cashews, oats, turkey. Fresh fruits and vegetables, also lightly steamed.

VITAMINS AND MINERALS—Vitamins A, B, C, D, and E. All help nourish and clean the veins. Calcium and magnesium, potassium, Silicon, copper, chromium, zinc.

HERBAL COMBINATIONS—Blood Purifier, Chelation, Digestion, Heart, Lower Bowel, Potassium.

SINGLE HERBS—Key Herbs: Capsicum, Garlic (antibiotic), Bugleweed, Burdock, Butcher's Broom, Dandelion, Ginkgo (improves circulation), Gotu Kola, Hops, Hawthorn (cleans veins), Kelp, Oatstraw (cleans veins), Rose Hips, Saffron (helps the body utilize fats), Suma. Other herbs: Black Cohosh, Lobelia, Blessed Thistle, Cramp Bark, Mistletoe, Parsley, Passion Flower, Scullcap, St. John's Wort, Valerian, Wood Betony, Yarrow, Yucca.

SUPPLEMENTS—Lecithin, Evening Primrose Oil, Salmon Oil, Blue-green algae, L-Carnitine, Co Q10, Germanium.

AVOID—Smoking, high fat diets, constipation, stress, caffeine, chocolate, sugar products.

CATARRH

(mucus)

This is an over-production of mucus in the respiratory system. Some call it a cold that has continued long enough to become chronic, such as in running nose, sinus problems, hay fever, allergies, cough, colds, tonsillitis, or earaches. People with catarrhal conditions are susceptible to all kinds of diseases. Catarrh is caused by the consumption of too many carbohydrates, sugars, starches and milk. It is aggravated by constipation. It starts in the stomach and can spread to the sinuses, tonsils, nasal cavities, ears, throat, bronchi and lungs.

Natural elimination must follow or many diseases can develop because germs and viruses seek the toxic waste and catarrh. Symptoms of catarrh include: "hacking cough", a dry throat, bad breath, itching ears, sore eyes, upset stomach, gas, shortness of breath, constipation or diarrhea.

NATURAL THERAPY—Fasting using lemon water (lemon has astringent and antiseptic properties), citrus juices, herbs and vegetable broths. Rest and chiropractic adjustments speed circulation for healing. Enema using catnip tea is good for children as well as for adults. Use an herbal laxative tea before going to bed; it will also bring fevers down quickly.

FOODS TO HEAL—Garlic, onions (soak in hot water and drink the juice). Vegetable broth with the following: potato peelings, onions, parsley, garlic, celery, carrots and tops, chives, and watercress.

VITAMINS AND MINERALS—A (essential for healthy mucus membranes), B-complex vitamins (depleted in acute diseases). C with bioflavonoids (necessary to prevent and heal catarrh conditions). All minerals are needed to prevent catarrh conditions. Calcium and magnesium, builds blood and sustains nerves. Potassium, sodium, selenium and zinc.

HERBAL COMBINATIONS—Allergy, Comfrey and Fenugreek (heals and breaks up mucus), Colds and Flu formulas, Infection, Lower Bowel, Nerves and Potassium.

SINGLE HERBS—Alfalfa-mint tea, Boneset (relieves pain and fevers), Capsicum, Comfrey (heals respiratory infections), Echinacea (cleansing and healing), Elder Flowers (cleans mucus), Fenugreek (loosens hardened mucous), Garlic (natural antibiotic), Ginger (settles stomach), Golden Seal (heals infections), Licorice, Lobelia (works with other herbs to heal), Marshmallow (soothes and heals catarrh conditions), Ma Hueng, Mullein (heals lungs), Passion Flower (relaxer), Peppermint (settles stomach), Rose Hips (rich in vitamin C and B-vitamins), Slippery Elm (provides protein for healing and heals throat and coughs).

SUPPLEMENTS—Acidophilus, Aloe Vera Juice, Liquid Chlorophyll, Blue-green Algae, Liquid Herbal and Mineral Supplement, Germanium, CO Q10.

AVOID—Mucus-forming foods such as milk, cheese, meat, bread, sugar, white flour products, pastries. Poor food combinations, such as eating starches with protein, or sugar with starches or protein. Overeating interferes with proper digestion and assimilation. Stress: learn how to handle stress in your life, only you can control stress.

CELIAC DISEASE
(gluten intolerance)

This is a relatively uncommon disorder which is found in some people as a genetic weakness, and in others it is seen as an environmental factor. One theory is when ingesting gluten it may trigger a preexisting immunologic response in a genetically susceptible person. Another theory is that a person with celiac disease may have an enzyme defect that causes an inability to digest gluten. This results in tissue toxicity as well as damage and weakness to the surface membranes of the small bowel.

Symptoms of celiac disease may include diarrhea, large and frequently foul-smelling stools that float, anemia, skin rash, nausea, abdominal distention due to flatulence, stomach cramps, weakness and weight loss.

NATURAL THERAPY—Prevent further irritation by eliminating gluten foods from the diet. Wheat, barley, rye and oats are the highest in gluten. Read food labels carefully to be certain that they do not contain gluten. The intestinal lining of the small intestine is damaged and has lost its ability to absorb essential nutrients. The loss of vital minerals and vitamins can cause serious problems.

FOODS TO HEAL—Carrots, apricots, sweet potatoes, sprouts, fertile eggs, yellow fruits and vegetables, raw goats milk, blackstrap molasses, legumes, green leafy vegetables, almonds, beans, root vegetables, sunflower seeds, berries, avocados, potatoes.

VITAMINS AND MINERALS—Vitamins A, D, K and E may be deficient because of the inability to absorb fat. B vitamins, C and iron are depleted quickly with diarrhea. All minerals must be supplemented, especially calcium and magnesium.

HERBAL COMBINATIONS—Blood Purifier, Anemia, Digestion, Bone.

SINGLE HERBS—Alfalfa, Burdock (blood cleanser), Dandelion, Kelp, Papaya, Psyllium (cleans the pockets of the colon), Saffron (digest oils), Slippery Elm (healing and high in protein), Yellow Dock.

SUPPLEMENTS—Chlorophyll, Blue-green algae, Glucomannan (cleans colon), Acidophilus, flaxseed tea. Essential fatty acids.

AVOID—Wheat, oats, barley and rye. Sugar (depletes nutrients), white flour products. Fried foods. Too much oil.

CHEMICAL IMBALANCE

Chemical imbalance is not a specific disease but has been implicated in persons who are depressed and mentally disturbed.

It is any condition which changes a normal pattern or chemical reactions the body goes through.

The activities of the brain that control our emotions are a set of chemicals called neurotransmitters. These may be unbalanced when the rest of the body seems healthy. The brain is extremely sensitive. In autointoxication, the brain suffers extreme toxic effects when the body seems strong in some other areas, and this condition will alter the functions of neurotransmitters.

Evaluating nutritional requirements is necessary for understanding what the body needs when an imbalance is present. A healthy liver is essential for a healthy brain. The liver is responsible for regulating hormones. It eliminates blood levels of estradiol, which is the "unfavorable" type of estrogen. If estradiol is allowed to enter the bloodstream, it can travel to the brain and cause depression and bizarre mental manifestations.

The one natural source to help chemical reactions in the brain is wholesome food. The brain is the seat of our emotions and is an organ of the body which needs nutrients, just as much as the liver or heart .

Intestinal toxemia cannot be overlooked in cases of depression, mental illness, or other types of brain dysfunction. In the early 1900's many medical doctors diagnosed toxemia, (self-poisoning) as the major cause of illness. Dr. Henry A. Cotton was one doctor who was involved with performing autopsies on mentally ill patients. He found that every one of the colons of those he examined had one or more problems. The bacterial poisons eventually act on the nerve supply of the abdominal organs, (causing spastic colitis). They also contribute to the production of atony and atrophy of the bowel walls; resulting in delayed motility, constipation and stasis. The ileoecal valve soon ceases to function normally and ileal stasis follows.

NATURAL THERAPY—In order to change the imbalance of the body, and to eliminate symptoms and to help the body heal itself, we need to activate chemical responses that adjust conditions back to a more desirable state of balance. Blood Purification and Lower Bowel cleansing are necessary to eliminate the toxins from traveling to the brain. The nerves need to be fed and strengthened.

FOODS TO HEAL—Whole grain (thermos cooking) to retain the B-vitamins and the enzymes for health. Millet, buckwheat, brown rice are excellent food. Raw and lightly steamed vegetables, fruits are health building. Sprouts and herbs to replace the elements that cause an imbalance.

VITAMINS AND MINERALS—B vitamins are essential for brain function. Vitamins A, C and E and the mineral selenium boost energy in the brain. Lecithin is necessary for proper brain function. All minerals are essential for proper body function.

HERBAL COMBINATIONS—Blood Purifiers, Bone, Digestion, Immune, Lower Bowels, Nerve, Stress.

SINGLE HERBS—Key Herbs: Ginkgo (antioxidant and increases circulation in the brain), Gotu Kola (feeds and nourishes the brain), Suma (provides oxygen to the brain), Dong Quai (blood cleanser), Ginseng (fortifies the whole body), Golden Seal (eliminates toxins), Hops (strengthens the nerves), Licorice (provides energy and feeds the glands), Passion Flower (relaxer for the nerves). Other herbs to benefit: Alfalfa, Black Cohosh, Black Walnut, Burdock, Capsicum, Chaparral, Dandelion, Ephedra, Echinacea, Garlic, Ginger, Hawthorn, Ho Shou-Wu, Lady's Slipper, Lobelia, Psyllium, Red Raspberry, Red Clover, Sarsaparilla, Scullcap, Yellow Dock.

SUPPLEMENTS—Bee Pollen, Spirulina, Chlorophyll, Evening Primrose Oil, Salmon Oil, Co-Q10, Germanium, Blue-green algae.

AVOID—Constipation, caffeine drinks, smoking, alcohol, chocolate, sugar products. Fried foods cause free radicals which lower the immune system.

CHEMICAL TOXICITY

Chemical additives and environmental toxins are a real health hazard. Our only defense is to strengthen our immune system. We need to be concerned about the water we drink, the food we eat and the air we breathe. Radioactive isotopes are invisible, odorless and tasteless and radiation of any kind is cumulative. Strontium 90 is very prevalent. Scientists say that everyone has potentially dangerous amounts of radioactive strontium in their bones. This can cause leukemia, sarcoma of the bones(bone cancer), Hodgkins disease, anemia, and weakness in the immune system.

One our greatest threats is plutonium, created from nuclear plants. We have tons of nuclear waste stored in the United States.

This waste is blown in the air, dumped in our soil, and filters in our water. It can cause lung cancer, leukemia, lymphoma and myeloma and cancer of the testes and ovaries.

Herbicide and pesticide residue are everywhere. We are constantly be exposed, and is found in the blood of persons living in both urban and rural areas. These poisons are capable of causing mutations and cancer. Lindane (bug bombs) is one example. It is used in home gardens, and on farms for fruits and vegetables and is a highly hazardous product. It is also used to treat seeds and hardwood lumber, and is popular in animal shampoos, flea collars, shelf paper and floor wax. It can cause cancer, is toxic to a growing fetus, damaging to reproductive organs, toxic to fish, and children are very susceptible.

Chemical additives in our food are numerous and have tripled in the past twenty years. Americans eat about ten pounds of chemical food additives a year. They are put in the seeds before they are planted, on the crops as they grow, and on the food as they are shipped to the consumer.

NATURAL THERAPY—Learn to read labels. Frozen food has a large amount of preservatives and additives. Learn to demand organically grown food, which is becoming more popular than ever before. Eat a balanced diet using more alkaline foods than acid. Keep the bowels in good working order and the bloodstream pure and clean.

FOODS TO HEAL-Raw or lightly steamed vegetables. Vegetable salads using sprouts (alfalfa, radish, fenugreek) and other vegetables.

Fruit is cleansing to the body. Eat whole grains cooked in a thermos or slow cooking in low heat to preserve enzymes.

Beans are a natural protection against built-up chemicals.

VITAMINS AND MINERALS—Vitamins A, D & E protect the immune system. Vitamin C with bioflavonoids protects the veins and immune system. B-complex protects the nerves. Multi-minerals, with extra calcium, selenium and zinc.

HERBAL COMBINATIONS—Blood Purifier, Bone, Chelation, Digestion, Immune, Lower Bowels, Glands.

SINGLE HERBS—Key Herbs: Bugleweed, Chaparral (cleans and eliminates toxins), Echinacea (blood cleanser), Garlic (neutralizes acids), Horseradish (antibiotic properties), Kelp (attracts chemical and moves them out of the body), Pau D'Arco (cleans blood and protects liver), Psyllium (cleans and removes toxins), Red Clover (blood purifier), Yellow Dock. Other beneficial herbs: Alfalfa, Aloe Vera, Comfrey, Fenugreek, Horsetail, Dulse, Ginkgo, Suma.

SUPPLEMENTS—Blue-green Algae, Chlorophyll, Pectin, Wheat Grass, Hydro-chloric Acid is essential in the blood to fight chemicals, infections, worms and parasites and to maintain the acid-alkaline balance. Salmon oil.

AVOID—Sugar (one cause of breaking down the immune system). The lungs breathe in chemicals: avoid sprays and toxins if possible.

Avoid fried foods, high meat diet, refined starches, salt, and high fat diet.

CHILDHOOD DISEASES

Germs cannot exist in a healthy and clean body. Childhood diseases are a cleansing and healing of a child's body from inherited or acquired weaknesses. Germs are nature's scavengers and can live only on weak cells, toxins in the body, and excess mucus.

If a child has a good strong body he will not get the childhood diseases. When children have access to sugar products, and use them day in and day out, this weakens the body and invites germs to feed off the toxins. Sugar is the downfall of the American diet; it leaches and weakens the body of nutrients that are vital for a healthy body. Processed food is void of minerals, vitamins and natural fiber essential for a healthy immune system.

Childhood diseases include chicken pox, measles, mumps, rubella (German Measles), rheumatic fever, scarlet fever and whooping cough. During chicken pox avoid aspirin, it could cause Reyes Syndrome. Measles causes a skin rash, and can lead to complications such as pneumonia and other lung, ear and eye infections. Mumps is a contagious viral infection and can spread to the ovaries, pancreas, testicles and the nervous system. Rheumatic fever is a strep infection and can affect the brain, heart and joints. Scarlet fever is a strep infection with sore throat, swollen lymph glands and cough. Scarlatina is a mild form of scarlet fever.

NATURAL THERAPY—Childhood diseases should be taken seriously and treated naturally. Keep the child warm and dry. Give plenty of liquids, especially citrus juices. Complications can follow childhood diseases if not treated properly. Vegetable broths will help. Use plenty of pure water. For fever, sponging with cold tap water will help bring it down. Avoid bright lights. Be alert for warning signs such as a high fever, delirium, listlessness, chest pains and breathing problems.

FOODS TO HEAL—Citrus juices diluted with pure water. Barley water with slippery elm bark will nourish and soothe the digestive tract, especially when diarrhea is present. Fasting is the best method so the liver can eliminate the toxins. Green drinks are cleansing. Wheat grass juice is also healing and cleansing.

VITAMINS AND MINERALS—Vitamin A is healing for the lungs and mucus membranes, B-complex vitamins depletes quickly in illness, Vitamin C with bioflavonoids will heal and help eliminate the toxins. Minerals are depleted fast in fevers and illness, extra calcium and magnesium, potassium selenium and zinc.

HERBAL COMBINATIONS—Colds and Flu combinations, Blood Purifier, Bone(extra calcium and minerals). Immune, Insomnia and Pain, Lower Bowel.

SINGLE HERBS—Key herbs: Catnip (acts as a sedative), Chamomile (calming for the nerves), Echinacea (cleans lymphatics and blood), Elder flowers (reduces fever along with peppermint), Garlic (natural antibiotic), Ginger (soothes stomach cramps), Golden Seal (very strong antibiotic, kills worms), Hops (relaxes nerves), Lobelia (relaxant and removes obstructions), Mullein, Pau D'Arco (blood cleanser), Peppermint (use after vomiting to calm stomach), Red Clover (blood cleanser), Rose Hips (rich in vitamin C and B-complex), Slippery Elm, Yarrow. Other herbs are Alfalfa, Capsicum, Cascara Sagrada (cleans bowels), Eyebright, Lady's Slipper, Pleurisy Root, Red Raspberry (soothing in fevers), Safflower, Scullcap, Yellow Dock.

SUPPLEMENTS—Chlorophyll, Aloe Vera Juice, Instant Vitamin C drinks.

AVOID—Stop eating food, for the liver and stomach are overburdened with eliminating the toxins to digest food. Sweets, alcohol, tobacco, chocolate,meat, and any food that interferes with healing. Stay away from drugs because this overstimulates the body. Remember natural healing takes its time, mother nature cannot be rushed.

CIRCULATION PROBLEMS
(Cold hands and feet)

The circulatory system consists of the heart, arteries, veins, and lymphatics. They serves as the body's transport system, bringing life-supporting oxygen and nutrients to cells, removing toxic waste, and carrying hormones from one part of the body to another.

Poor circulation is seen in the extremities of the hands, fingers, feet, toes, the head, the nose and genitals. Poor circulation is felt by cold fingers and toes, cold nose, tingling feelings in the extremities, muscle aches, impotency in male, frigidity in the female, dry eyes, (or any other mucus membrane), ringing of the ears, dizziness or mental alertness, irritability and insomnia.

Blood circulates through the arteries, veins and capillaries. The blood carries nutrients to all parts of the body but it also can carry toxins to any organ or part of the body. Autointoxication can cause the blood to carry toxins that will accumulate in the veins and interfere with proper blood circulation. This can cause cold hands and feet. When the blood is overloaded with toxins circulation becomes impaired.

Insufficient supply of blood is seen in diabetes, accumulation of plaque on the inner lining of the blood vessels and stress. The nervous system when under stress inhibits complete blood vessel dilation. Poor blood circulation is created.

NATURAL THERAPY—Blood Purification, Skin Brushing along with hot and cold showers. Deep breathing exercises Exercise will help increase circulation. Learn to control stress, it is a factor in constriction of vessels and poor circulation. A common sense approach to circulatory problems would be to create a natural nutitional program to prevent further accumulation of plaque, dissolving particles already present and to clean the arteries of material to provide for better circulation.

FOODS TO HEAL—Eat a high fiber diet. Oat bran will help in circulation by lowering cholesterol levels. Bananas, broccoli, brown rice, millet, beans, peas, a lot of green salads with lots of raw vegetables. Citrus juices, vegetables juices such as carrot, beet, celery, parsley. Green vegetables are blood cleansers. Green drinks using wheat grass, sprouts, parsley, comfrey leaves.

VITAMINS AND MINERALS—Vitamins A, D and E are essential for a healthy circulatory system. Niacinamide-niacin (deficiency can result in depression, sleeplessness, body aches and irritability), and B-complex vitamins increases circulation and reduces cholesterol levels. Vitamin B6, removes excess water in the tissues (poor circulation can be due to water excess). Vitamin C with bioflavonoids are necessary for healthy veins, especially the capillaries. Choline and inositol (found in lecithin). Multi-mineral with extra selenium and zinc (helps in glandular problems, anemia and in insomnia. Magnesium along with vitamin D is necessary for calcium assimilation. It removed excess calcium from the blood stream.

HERBAL COMBINATIONS—Blood Purifier, Chelation, Digestion, Heart, Potassium.

SINGLE HERBS—Key herbs: Hawthorn (nourishes the heart and veins), Capsicum (increases circulation and cleans the veins), Lobelia, Garlic (lowers cholesterol), Bugleweed (equalizes circulation), Burdock (blood cleanser), Butcher's Broom (improves circulation to prevent blood clots), Ephedra, Ginseng, Gotu Kola (improves brain circulation), Horsetail (strengthens immune system), Mistletoe (constrict blood vessels), Parsley (natural diuretic), Psyllium (cleans colon of toxins), Prickly Ash (increases circulation in cold extremities and joints), Scullcap. Other herbs: Black Cohosh, Blessed Thistle, Cramp Bark, Dandelion, Hops, Kelp, Lily of the Valley, Oatstraw, Passion Flower, Rose Hips, Saffron, St. Johnswort, Valerian, Wood Betony, Yarrow.

SUPPLEMENTS—Chlorophyll (rebuilds heart), Lecithin (prevents and dissolves fatty deposits), Flaxseeds, Evening Primrose Oil, Fish Oil Lipids, Salmon Oil (dissolves fatty deposits in the blood), Glucomannan, Rice Bran Syrup. Co Q10, Germanium, L-Carnitine, Apple pectin (lowers cholesterol and regulates bowel function).

AVOID—Coffee, tea, cola or other caffeinated beverages, alcoholic drinks, and smoking. These cause circulation problems. High meat diet produces uric acid, and toxins. Constipation will cause toxins to accumulate in the blood and create poor circualation.

Avoid fatty and greasy foods, sugar, salt and hydrogenated oils. Fats clog up the lymphatic system and slows the natural eliminatory system.

COLITIS
(diverticulosis)

Colitis is inflammation of the colon which causes loose and watery stools, often containing mucus, diarrhea and bleeding from the rectum. There can be alternate constipation and diarrhea, incomplete emptying of the bowels, and pain. Other symptoms are indigestion, headaches, fatigue and distension. It is a disease of the large intestine and affects an estimated 250,000 people in the United States.

There are different types of colitis, which can be mild or serious. Inflammation of the small intestine such as enteritis and ileitis are associated with colitis. In severe cases there can be anemia, weight loss, fever and a tender, bloated stomach.

NATURAL THERAPY—Healing therapy using demulcent herbs. Enemas or colonics clean the bowels. Use mild food until healing takes place. Using nervine herbal therapy will speed healing. A change in diet and life style will eventually stabilize peristaltic movements and remove irritation. Worry, tension and fatigue can put a burden on the colon.

FOODS TO HEAL—A few days fasting using carrot juice and demulcent herb teas like comfrey, mullein and slippery elm,. Steamed carrots, potatoes, squash. Avocados, eggplant, bananas. Grated fresh apples, pears and peaches. Avoid the skin until healing takes place. Put steamed or raw vegetables into a blender. Add psyllium or oat bran to liquids.

VITAMINS AND MINERALS—Vitamin A (heals mucus membranes), Vitamin C and bioflavonoids (builds the immune system), Vitamin E for tissue healing, Vitamin B Complex (necessary for health and digestion), Mineral supplement (lost in diarrhea) also essential for healing. Calcium, and magnesium, chromium and zinc. Also silicon and selenium. Deficiency of vitamin A, E, and K are common in colitis.

HERBAL COMBINATIONS—Bone and Potassium, Ulcer, Digestion and Lower Bowels. Nervine herbs help in all healing.

SINGLE HERBS—Aloe Vera (very healing), Alfalfa (contains vitamin K), Dandelion, Garlic, Hops, Kelp, Lobelia, Marshmallow, Myrrh, Papaya, Pau D'Arco, Psyllium, Scullcap, Slippery Elm, Yellow Dock.

SUPPLEMENTS—Acidophilus (milk free), Liquid Chlorophyll, Salmon Oil, or Evening Primrose Oil, Glucomannan (before meals), Blue-green Algae.

AVOID—Over-the-counter laxatives (only irritates more), sugar, and other refined carbohydrates, insufficient chewing of food. Avoid emotional conflicts. Stress is an aggravating factor in colitis. Avoid fried food, condiments and excessive amounts of dairy products, chocolate, and caffeine drinks. Smoking, fumes and chemical sprays, and toxic food additives.

CONSTIPATION

The American diet which is lacking in fiber is the main reason for constipation. The lack of fiber causes the food to remain too long a time in the colon and causes bacteria and toxins to accumulate. The longer food is retained means more water is absorbed, leaving the waste material dry, hard and difficult to evacuate. Under normal conditions the colon produces mucus to protect the intestinal wall, which keeps the material moving at a regular and smooth pace. But with constipation the colon loses its natural mucus when the water is absorbed, and the feces attach themselves directly to the intestinal wall. This builds up over the years with a high fat and white flour diet, which is like putting paste- or glue-like substances on the colon walls. This creates chronic diseases, and unless it is eliminated can cause cancer and other life threatening ailments.

Bowel constipation over the years can back up poisons into the venous, arterial and lymphatic systems, and enter every cell of the body. Old fecal matter will balloon the bowel and weaken it, allowing bacterial toxins to enter the blood stream. The toxins then poison the nerves surrounding the colon, ultimately affecting all other related tissues, organs and systems.

Autointoxication is the result of constipation and a process whereby the body poisons itself by harboring a cesspool of decaying matter in the colon. It contains a high concentration of harmful bacteria. The toxins released by the decaying food gets into the bloodstream and goes to all parts of the body and weakens the entire system.

The ileocecal valve can become incompetent and cause regurgitation into the small intestine, which contain dangerous poisons to be reabsorbed into the blood stream. The incompetency of this valve is believed to be due to the enlargement of the cecum pulling the valve apart and preventing its closure.

The endocrine glands cannot handle the toxic load when the colon is backed up, and it becomes congested and unable to perform hundreds of functions vital to the health of the body.

People who are constipated, and don't eliminate after every meal, could have several days or weeks of waste matter in their colon.

NATURAL THERAPY—Lower Bowel Cleansing and Blood Purification is necessary. Colonics may be necessary to loosen the encrusted colon. Drink plenty of fresh fruit and vegetable juices. Exercise is essential for a healthy colon. Food combining and chewing food properly are vital to prevent constipation. Eat high fiber foods.

Sit-ups or slant board (poor muscle tone is usually present when constipation exists, causing pockets to form in the intestines, holding partially digested food). Deep breathing (oxygen is essential for respiration of all cells to detoxify waste material, which lack of can cause free radical formation and premature aging.

The colon is the principal organ for the detoxification of the lymph glands. Rebound exercises helps remove toxins from the lymph glands. Skin brushing promotes elimination.

FOODS TO HEAL—Fresh lemon juice in water first thing in the morning will help. Molasses, yogurt, wheat germ and bran. Soaked prunes, figs and raisins. Raw beet, carrot and celery juices. Apples, peaches, berries, oranges. Sprouted seed, grains and nuts. Eat whole grains like millet, whole wheat, barley, buckwheat, oats, corn meal. Raw vegetable salads are an excellent way to add nutrition and bulk. Beans and lentils. Almond and sesame seed milk drinks lubricate the bowels.

VITAMINS AND MINERALS—Vitamins A (a steady supply to strengthen and repair the tissues), Vitamin C and bioflavonoids (to control the sievability of the cells. B-Complex, D, E (too much fat can cause deficiency of vitamin E), and K. Multi-minerals (liquid), calcium and magnesium, selenium, zinc, silicon will help the absorption of calcium and other minerals. Iron deficiency may be related to toxins and poor elimination.

HERBAL COMBINATIONS—Blood Purifier, Digestion, Immune, Liver and Gall Bladder, Lower Bowel, and Red Clover Blends.

SINGLE HERBS—Herbs have the ability to loosen hard material from the colon. Aloe Vera, Alfalfa, Barberry, Buckthorn, Burdock, Cascara Sagrada (cleans and rebuilds colon), Comfrey, Dandelion, Fennel, Fenugreek (loosens hard mucus), Ginger, Golden Seal, Kelp, Licorice, Mullein, Myrrh, Pau D' Arco, Psyllium, (excellent for removing loosened material). It swells when taken with water, forming a bulky residue and has the ability to absorb large quantities of sticky, gluey material along the colon walls). Senna (keeps colon clean), Slippery Elm (heals and nourishes colon), Yarrow.

SUPPLEMENTS—Apple Pectin, Acidophilus, Chlorophyll, Flaxseed, Wheat Grass, Bentonite, Fiber Cookie.

AVOID—Refined foods that cause constipation. Avoid laxatives; they are dangerous and habit forming. They interfere with the proper absorption of critically vital sodium and potassium balance in the large intestine. Potassium is lost when laxatives are taken. Herbal laxatives rebuild, heal and provide nutrients for a healthy colon. Dairy products are mucus-forming and constipating. Avoid mineral oil. It depletes vitamin A and other vitamins from the body. Avoid chemicals, additives and junk food which stress the body's ability to digest. Antibiotics destroy the bacterial flora in the colon.

CROHN'S DISEASE

There are an ever-increasing number of people who are becoming afflicted with the disorder known as "Crohn's Disease." It is alarming, because this disease, which affects the gastrointestinal tract, is very serious. It is an inflammation of any portion of the GI tract, and extends through all layers of the intestinal wall.

The disease is characterized by scarring and narrowing of the colon, due to inflammation, and sometimes it is so severe that the colon becomes blocked and nothing can pass through. There is a lot of pain associated with this disease, which is often first manifested by diarrhea, weight loss, low stress tolerance, abdominal infections and anemia.

It is felt that Crohn's disease is an "autoimmune" disorder. It may be that the entire body (especially the gastrointestinal tract) becomes so toxic from many years of toxin buildup from medications, poor eating habits, etc., that the immune system becomes confused. It then attacks the toxic tissues, and begins to destroy them, thinking they are a foreign organism.

Many nutritionsts feel that there is extreme parasite infestation associated with this disease. This further debilitates the immune system, of which Crohn's disease victims are already weak. An overburdened lymphatic system is another cause. High stress seems to be a factor. Young people (twelve years of age) are coming down with it. This indicates that maybe the mother's prenatal diet and postnatal diet for the child could be a factor.

NATURAL THERAPY—A nutritional approach would be to Cleanse, Eliminate parasites, work with digestion and build the immune system. Blood Purification and Colon Healing Therapies. Drink plenty of liquids, pure water, herbal teas, fresh juices, Wheat grass juice is healing. Watch food combining. Juice fasts are very healing. Add other foods after healing of the colon takes place.

FOODS TO HEAL—Blend fresh and steamed vegetables and chew well food such as broccoli, brussels sprouts, carrots, celery, cabbage, kale, spinach. Herbs are very healing and provide vitamins and minerals and are considered food. Slippery Elm is a food and will heal the colon. Use thermos cooking for delicious mush. Pour boiling water over whole grains, and let stand over night. Millet is easy to digest. Vegetable broths are healing and rich in minerals.

VITAMIN AND MINERALS—Vitamins A and C are healing for the immune system. Bioflavonoids are necessary with the vitamin C. B-Complex vitamins are necessary for proper digestion. B-Vitamin deficiencies and poor absorption of nutrients are the major nutritional problems. Vitamin E along with A, and C, help control infections. Multi-vitamin and mineral supplements are essential; deficiency is common in Crohn's disease. Selenium and zinc are also very healing. Vitamin K supplement is necessary.

HERBAL COMBINATIONS—Anemia, Glands, Digestion, Immune, Potassium, Lower Bowel, Ulcer.

SINGLE HERBS-Aloe Vera (healing), Alfalfa (provides all minerals), Dandelion, Garlic, Hops, Kelp, Lobelia, Marshmallow, Myrrh, Papaya, Pau D'Arco, Psyllium (healing and cleansing for the colon), Saffron (helps in the assimilation of oils), Scullcap (repairs nerves), Slippery Elm (food for the colon), Yellow Dock.

SUPPLEMENTS—Digestive enzymes. Essential Fatty Acids, such as Salmon Oil, Evening Primrose Oil, Acidophilus (provides friendly bacteria in colon), Liquid Chlorophyll, Glucomannan, Flax Seed drink.

AVOID—Meat is hard on the digestive system, especially beef and pork. Sugar and all sugar products deplete essential nutrients. Avoid soft drinks, chocolate, candy, cookies, cakes, all pastry products. Avoid caffeine, drugs and all products that lowers the immune system.

COLDS, FLU, AND FEVERS

Colds, flu and fevers are part of nature's natural eliminative process, a safety valve which the body opens of its own accord to give the body the chance for a natural process to take place. If we use the drugs to suppress the flu or colds, that which should have been eliminated is retained within the body. As long as we continue to suppress the natural process of elimination the toxic material begins to settle in the organs of the body to eventually create what we call chronic disease such as arthritis, diabetes, chronic asthma, etc.

Modern medical science's theory is to kill the germ and cure the disease. It has developed drug therapy that suppresses the acute diseases and either complicates the disease or throws it deeper into the organs to cause a chronic disease later.

All acute diseases are based on Nature's Law or Cure. Scientists all around the world have been seeking for a cure to eliminate the common cold. They will never find a cure for acute diseases, for they are the cure.

Natural methods create a positive effect on the health of the whole body. If drugs are the method chosen to treat acute diseases, the body is hindered in its ability to eliminate the toxins and causes them to remain in the body, usually in the weakest part.

Fever speeds up the body's healing process. The heart beats faster, the liver increases its acitvity destroying more toxins, the kidney's excrete more acids to clean the blood, the glandular system produces more hormones for normal body function and the body cells produce more interferons to fight illness.

NATURAL THERAPY—Cleansing the colon, and Blood Purification will help eliminate the toxins. Stop eating; the body is trying to squeeze out the toxins and dump them in the stomach. When eating the healing and cleansing has to stop to digest the food. Use herbal teas and citrus juices for cleansing the body. A lot of rest is necessary for healing.

FOODS TO HEAL—Citrus juices with herbal teas are the most healing. Vegetable broths will strengthen the system.

VITAMINS AND MINERALS—Vitamin A heals and protects the immune system. Vitamin C (with bioflavonoids), heals and destroys germs and viruses. B Vitamins are needed during illness. Multi-mineral supplement is needed for all healing and to maintain nutritionl balance. Selenium and zinc are healing. Calcium and magnesium are healing. Potassium is lost during illness, supplement is necessary.

HERBAL COMBINATIONS—Allergy, Cold and Flu, Infection, Lower Bowel, Nerves, and Potassium.

SINGLE HERBS—Alfalfa and mint tea, Aloe Vera, Capsicum, Comfrey, Dandelion, Fenugreek, Garlic, Ginger (settles stomach), Golden Seal, Kelp (provides minerals and heals), Licorice, Lobelia, Marshmallow, Mullein, Passion Flower, Red Raspberry, Rose Hips, Slippery Elm (for coughs and heals throat).

SUPPLEMENTS—Aloe Vera juice, liquid chlorophyll, Blue-green Algae.

AVOID—Eating solid food, meat, grains, sugar, sweet fruit juices until healing takes place.

COUGHS

Coughing is a protective reflex, aimed at ridding the body of mucus, air pollution or irritants in the breathing apparatus. They vary in nature and severity. Some coughs are just a tickle in the throat that lasts for a few days and some are coughs that develop from a cold into bronchitis, pneumonia, asthma, tuberculosis or even cancer of the lungs. When a cough lasts more than a few weeks care must be taken to look at the whole body and do some cleansing.

Poisons and toxins in the body make one susceptible to coughs, cold, flu and acute diseases. A low alkaline diet lowers resistance. Improper diet, as well as a lack of fresh air and exercise lowers vitality. Air pollution puts an extra burden on the lungs and lowers resistance to an already lowered system.

Different kinds of coughs are croupy, or hard, feverish, watery, catarrhal (phlegm), and chronic. Croupy cough usually comes on suddenly with a loud rasping sound and the phlegm is difficult to cough up, and the child usually sounds worse than it really is. This cough is caused by inflammation of the larynx and trachea, with hardened and thick phlegm. A feverish cough comes on suddenly and is caused by an infection. If it is bronchitis the chest is tight and painful.A watery cough is usually caused from the nose draining down the throat. It is usually brought on during cold, wet weather when there is a lowered immune system. A catarrhal cough usually accompanies infections. It is worse when lying down, the cough produces thick, white phlegm, or thick white or green phlegm from the nose. It usually accompanies a cold. Chronic coughs are brought on because the initial cough was suppressed from eating with a cold or taking drugs for the cold. The mucus in the head area was never cleared out but was suppressed and hardened.

NATURAL THERAPY—Change the diet to eliminate mucus from the stomach. The stomach and bowels need to be cleansed to keep the system in good working order. Stress can cause toxins to accumulate and put an extra burden on the immune system. An over-all change of living habits needs to be evaluated.

FOODS TO HEAL—Citrus juices until the acute symptoms disappear. Vegetable broths, green drinks and herbal eas will help heal faster than eating food during acute disease.

VITAMINS AND MINERALS—Vitamin A (high amounts at first), C with bioflavonoids (1,000 mil every hour at first), B-complex (is depleted fast during illness). Calcium, magnesium, potassium, selenium and zinc.

HERBAL COMBINATIONS—Colds and Flu, Infection, Lower Bowel, Nerves, Potassium, Red Cover blend.

SINGLE HERBS—Key herbs: Alfalfa (tea), Aloe Vera (healing a prevent scar tissues), Comfrey (healing), Fenugreek (prevents mucus from forming and loosens hard mucus), Garlic (kills germs and heal infections), Ginger (settles stomach), Golden Seal (kills germs, viruses and parasites), Lobelia (removes obstructions), Marshmallow, Mullein, Red Raspberry, Rose Hips, Slippery Elm (for coughs and also heals throat and stomach). Other herbs: Capsicum, Dandelion, Kelp, Licorice, Ma Hueng, Passion Flower (soothing for nerves), Scullcap (feeds and heals nerves), Pau D'Arco (cleans and kill germs).

SUPPLEMENTS—Green drinks, Rice Bran syrup, Chinese essential oils (external), peppermint tea, tea tree oil. Liquid herbal extracts.

AVOID—Stop eating during acute disease. The stomach needs to eliminate the mucus and toxins to repair and heal the body. Avoid antibiotics and drugs which only suppress the coughs and drainage.

CYSTIC FIBROSIS

Cystic Fibrosis is a genetic disorder—a recessive genetic trait—which has to be carried by both parents to have an afflicted child. The chances of having an affected child with Cystic Fibrosis when both parents carry those recessive genes is 25 percent. Most people never realize that they are carriers of these recessive genetic traits until they have a child with Cystic Fibrosis. It is the most common fatal genetic disease of Caucasian children.

Cystic Fibrosis is a generalized dysfunction of the exocrine and endocrine systems in varying degrees of severity. The gastrointestinal effects of cystic fibrosis occur mainly in the intestines, pancreas and liver. One of the earliest such symptoms is 'meconium ileus'. The newborn with cystic fibrosis doesn't excrete meconium, a dark green mucilaginous material found in the intestine at birth. He develops symptoms of intestinal obstruction, such as abdominal distention, vomiting, constipation, dehydration and electrolyte imbalance. Eventually, obstruction of the pancreatic ducts and resulting deficiency of trypsin, amylase, and lipase prevent the conversion and absorption of fat and protein in the intestinal tract.

The undigested food is then excreted in frequent bulky, foul smelling and pale stools with a high fat content. The inability of the body to absorb nutrients produces poor weight gain, a ravenous appetite, sallow skin and distended abdomen. The inability to absorb fats produces deficiencies of the fat soluble vitamins (A, E, E, and K), leading to clotting problems and retarded bone growth.

NATURAL THERAPY—Blood Purification and Colon Cleansing Therapy are essential. Carrot juice mixed with celery, cucumber, then beet juice, all in small amounts with larger amounts of carrot juice. Diet is very important.

FOODS TO HEAL—Carrot juice with smaller amounts of beet, celery, cucumber. Wheat grass juice is healing and supplies protein and minerals and vitamins. Slippery Elm added to juices will heal and also supply protein. Other mild foods can be added as strength is gained and healing is improved. Raw foods are essential to supply nutrients.

VITAMINS AND MINERALS—Vitamin A to protect the mucus membranes and to prevent infections. Beta-carotene will absorb better. Vitamin A derived from carrot juice will also supply calcium. Vitamin E is needed (difficult to absorb); Vitamin C is essential to those with cystic fibrosis because they are always plagued with frequent infections. Small frequent doses work better. All minerals are essential; they are easily lost with diarrhea.

HERBAL COMBINATIONS—Anemia, Glands, Digestion, Immune, Lung, Lower Bowel.

SINGLE HERBS—Key herbs: Comfrey (healing), Fennel (for digestion), Ginger, Lady's Slipper (works on the medulla in the brain helping to regulate breathing, sweating, saliva and heart function). Lobelia, Marshmallow, Mullein, Papaya, Peppermint, Saffron (digests fats), Slippery Elm. Other helpful herbs: Pau D'Arco, Red Clover, Scullcap, Kelp, Dulse, and other sea weeds are nourishing.

SUPPLEMENTS—Acidophilus, Free-Form Amino Acids, Pancreatic Digestive Enzymes. Chlorophyll, Glucomannan (keeps colon clean), Salmon Oil, Evening Primrose Oil, Blue-green Algae.

AVOID—Processed food, meat, too much cooked food. Mucus forming foods. Because of defects in the organs a thick, clogging mucus draws infections and obstructs the lungs and intestines. Avoid drugs, antibiotics, aspirin.

CYSTS AND TUMORS

A cyst is a closed sac or pouch with a definite wall which contains fluid, semifluid or solid material. Tumors are a swelling or abnormal growth of tissues having no useful function in the body. Cancer cells are abnormal cells that invade healthy tissues. They travel through the system, and deposit themselves in the weakest areas of the body causing growths or tumors. Suppressing acute diseases are the cause of cysts and tumors. Mucus is allowed to accumulate and harden in the body when acute diseases are not allowed to go through the five stages of healing.

NATURAL THERAPY—Cleansing the blood and cells with short fasts, juices, and herbs to help loosen and eliminate the cysts and tumors.

FOODS TO HEAL—High fiber foods, deep yellow and dark green vegetables and fruits. Sweet potatoes, yams, squash, carrots, peaches, apricots.

VITAMINS AND MINERALS—Vitamin A (antioxidant, destroys free radicals), B-complex (repairs cells), C (heals and protects against cancer). Calcium, magnesium and potassium, selenium and zinc (protects the immune system).

HERBAL COMBINATIONS—Blood Purifier, Digestion, Immune, Lower Bowels, Nerves.

SINGLE HERBS—Burdock, Chaparral (cleans and dissolves cysts and tumors), Dandelion (cleans the liver), Echinacea (cleans the lymphatics), Garlic (kills germs), Golden Seal (kills and destroys germ and acts as an antibiotic), Kelp (very healing and cleansing), Milk Thistle (helps heal liver), Parsley, Pau D'Arco (purifies the blood), Prickly Ash (aids in circulation), Red Clover (Red Clover Blend Tea), Suma (strengthens the body), Yellow Dock.

SUPPLEMENTS—Acidophilus, Lecithin, Liquid Chlorophyll, Salmon Oil, Wheat Grass Juice, Fish Oil Lipids.

AVOID—Meat, white sugar, white flour products. Fried foods, Antibiotics (weakens the Immune System). Caffeine, alochol, chocolate, candy, cookies, pastries, all soft drinks. Avoid all food additives, and food colorings. Watch for sulfites and sulfates. Avoid smoking and using over the counter drugs.

DEPRESSION

Depression is common and widespread as the common cold or mental illness. Depression is a real affliction—it is not a sign of weakness. Neither is depression a hopeless condition. It can be treated nutritionally with successful results. The brain needs nutrition as much or more than the other organs of the body. The brain's neurotransmitters, which are responsible in regulating our behavior, are controlled by the diet we eat.

Depression was called melancholia in the past. Many doctors found that autointoxication was the main cause of depression and mental problems. The brain is very sensitive to toxins. When the bowels are not kept clean the toxins enter the blood and travel to the brain. One medical doctor wrote in an article in the Medical Record in 1937, speaking about the stagnant bowel which cannot be considered as normal on the criteria accepted today even with two or three bowel movements a day. "No matter how many stools or what their physical character may be, even if fluid, marked retention of toxic or sapremic substances may exist. Many of the most toxic individuals that I have seen have daily and often more frequent bowel movements."

The World Health Organization conducted a survey and found that 200 million persons worldwide suffer from depression. All of us face depression one time or another in one form or another. Stressful situations cause depression. Normal depression comes with grief as in a death, divorce, loss of job, medical problems or other stressful situations. A mild chronic depression, where the "blues" continue, there can be negative feelings and dissatisfaction with life. One loses interest in life, family and friends, and is often fatigue. There are also feelings of anger, anxiety and worthlessness.

Major depression can happen when one feels there is no relief in sight. There is usually change in sleeping habits. There is loss of appetite or some suffer from eating too much. The person may feel guilt and wish they were dead. They have feelings of anxiety, dread, worthlessness, and ill fate. This can also alternate with periods of normal behavior.

Manic depression is manifested by periods of high elation, working sprees, wild spending sprees, constant moving and action followed by deep depression.

Prozac is a popular, widely prescribed drug that doctors are using on three million people accross the country for depression. It was approved by the FDA in December 1987 and was reported as having few side effects. This is a drug to be very careful of because even the manufacturer admits that Prozac can cause agitation, hostility, psychosis, and other frightening side effects such as "akathidia". Information of warning about Prozac states the following possible adverse reactions: Nervous System: abnormal dreams and agitation; infrequent: abnormal gait, acute brain syndrome, akathisia, anmesia, apathy, delusions, depersonalization, euphoria, hallucinations, hositlity, manic reaction, paranoid reaction, psychosis and vertigo. Rare: abnormal electroencephalogram, anti-social reaction, chronic brain syndrome, and hysteria.

NATURAL THERAPY—Blood and Colon cleansing (clean blood for the brain). Toxins from the colon enter the blood stream and travel to the brain and cause all kinds of weird thinking. Build the nervous system with herbs, food and supplements. The circulatory system needs to be kept clean to supply oxygen and nutrients to the brain.

FOODS TO HEAL—Complex carbohydrates such as brown rice, millet, buckwheat, corn meal, wheat, oats (they contain tryptophan which has a calming effect). Protein creates alertness (contains dopamine and norepinephrine). Turkey breast (organically grown), high in tryptophan. Fish is high in protein, salmon, cod, and tuna are good. Beans (dry) are high in protein. Fresh and steamed vegetables are rich in minerals which are essential for the brain and nervous system.

VITAMINS AND MINERALS—Vitamin A, B-complex (with extra B6, B12, folic acid, niacin). Vitamin C and bioflavonoids (along with B6 are converted into brain neurotransmitter). Multi-minerals are essential for brain health. Extra calcium, magnesium, selenium and zinc.

HERBAL COMBINATIONS—Blood Purifier, Bone, Digestion, Immune, Lower Bowels, Potassium, Nerve and stress combinations.

SINGLE HERBS—Key herbs: Gotu Kola (brain food), Capsicum (blood circulation), Ginseng (energy food), Kelp (cleans glands and veins), Dong Quai (tranquilizing on nerves), Garlic (cleansing), Chamomile (rich in calcium to feed the nerves). Skullcap (rebuilds the nerves), Hops (sedative properties), Passion Flower (soothing on the nerves). Ginkgo (stimulates brain function), Suma (increases oxygen supply to the brain). Other beneficial herbs: Alfalfa, Black Cohosh, Black Walnut, Burdock, Chaparral, Dandelion, Ephedra, Echinacea, Ginger, Golden Seal, Hawthorn, Ho Shou-Wu, Lady's Slipper, Licorice, Lobelia, Red Raspberry, Red Clover, Wood Betony, Yellow Dock.

SUPPLEMENTS-Bee Pollen, Spirulina, Chlorophyll, Essential fatty acids such as Evening Primrose Oil, Salmon Oil. Blue-green Algae, Lecithin.

AVOID—Heavy metal poisoning (severe depression can be a symptom of lead poisoning, or other metals), Allergies can cause severe depression. Caffeine addiction creates thiamine deficiency and weakens the nervous system, and the lack of other B vitamins can cause depression. Avoid junk food as it puts a double stress on the body and dulls the appetite for wholesome food. Sugar throws the body out of balance, harms the pancreas and depletes the essential B vitamins and calcium from the body. Too much meat causes uric acid and other toxins to accumulate in the blood. Alcohol creates a lot of hard work for the detoxifying organs: liver, kidneys, pancreas, also depletes vitamins and minerals.

Constant stress will cause the nerves to weaken and put a burden on the glands and organs of the body. Learn stress management through relaxation, mediation, and exercise.

DIABETES

Diabetes is increasing at a fast rate , more than 10 million Americans have this disease. It is estimated that two out of five of them do not realize they have diabetes. Americans overeat too many fast foods. Diabetes is unknown in countries where people can't afford to overeat.People with diabetes are up to four times more likely to die from a heart attack. And people with diabetes are have a greater risk of having strokes.

Symptoms are excessive thirst and urination, and excessive hunger. General weakness and depression and skin disorders, including boils and vaginal infections, blurred vision, tingling leg cramps, impotence, and a dry mouth are frequent complaints.

There are two types of diabetes. The first is Type 1, Juvenile diabetes mellitus also called insulin dependent diabetes mellitus (IDDM). In this type the pancreas does not produce insulin, a hormone which delivers the glucose to the cells. Insulin is formed in the Islets of Langerhans, where it is responsible for moving the sugar in the blood and into the cells. This is a more serious diabetes and almost always develops in childhood.

In Type 2 diabetes the pancreas is producing insulin, but the cells have too few chemical receptors and the cells starve, resulting in lack of energy. The major cause of Type 2 is now thought to be obesity. Overeating and eating the wrong kinds of food are the major cause. It is like you are starving your body while eating a lot of food.

NATURAL THERAPY—Blood Purification, Bowel Cleansers through enemas, colonics or Lower Bowel cleansers. A change of diet. Sugar is the American diets' downfall. Sugar is put in our food, in canned, frozen and fast foods. A natural diet is very vital. Fasting will help eliminate sugar from the cells in the body. Short fasts are very important to prevent weakening the body before it is strong enough to handle long fasts. Exercise and skin brushing will speed the cleansing and healing of the body. Exercise helps the body use up excess blood sugar. Thirty to sixty minutes of aerobic exercise a day benefits the body up to twelve hours later.

A diet change is the biggest challenge a diabetic has. They don't want to change their eating habits.

FOODS TO HEAL—Sprouted grains added to salads and in vegetable casseroles. A lot of non-starchy vegetables, lightly steamed and drink the juice. Vegetables such as asparagus, green beans, okra, celery, watercress, parsley, alfalfa, jerusalem artichokes (a starch the pancreas can handle). Goat milk and whey powder are high in sodium. Sprouts (alfalfa, bean, radish and fenugreek), garlic, onions endive, fresh fruits and berries, beets, leafy green vegetables.

A high-fiber diet helps to lower blood triglycerides in diabetics and prediabetics. Fiber has the ability to repair faulty sugar metabolism by its complex effect on stomach and intestinal functioning. Psyllium hulls, grains such whole oats, wheat, millet, buckwheat, barley, brown rice.

VITAMINS AND MINERALS—A, use natural (beta-carotene is difficult for the diabetic to convert into vitamin A), protects the eyes from damage. All vitamins are involved directly or indirectly in maintaining normal sugar metabolism. B-complex vitamins help to cut down on insulin intake, strengthen and repair nerves. Vitamin C with bioflavo oids, essential for artery health, cleans the veins and strengthens the immune system. E necessary to help the body store sugar as glycogen. Helps iron to be absorbed by the thyroid, cuts down on artery complications. Amino acids are important: L-Carnitine and L-glutamine helps the liver to metabolize fat.

All minerals are essential for the diabetic. Chromium helps the body to stabilize blood sugar. Copper aids the body in utilizing enzymes and protein assimilation. Calcium is vital for the nerves when used along with magnesium to balance the body. Biotin and inositol, found in lecithin are essential for all body functions. Silicon is essential for cleaning the body to improve the health of diabetics. Zinc is on of the main ingredients of insulin. A lack is seen in diabetics. Potassium is necessary for the diabetic.

HERBAL COMBINATIONS—Blood Purifier, Bone, Lower Bowels, Pancreas and Diabetes, Parasites and Worms, Potassium and Stress.

SINGLE HERBS-Key herbs: Alfalfa, Aloe Vera, Black Walnut (kills parasites), Buchu, Burdock (cleans blood), Cedar Berries (heals the pancreas), Cornsilk, Dandelion, Garlic, Gentian, Golden Seal (acts as insulin, stops internal bleeding), Hawthorn, Horsetail, Kelp, Psyllium. Other beneficial herbs. Capsicum, Chaparral, Echinacea, Ginger, Ginseng, Irish Moss, Juniper Berries, Licorice, Lobelia, Myrrh, Parsley, Queen of the Meadow, Red Clover, Uva, Ursi, Watercress, Wormwood, Yellow Dock.

SUPPLEMENTS—Liquid Chlorophyll, Blue-green Algae, Lecithin, Glucomannan, Rice Bran Syrup, Salmon Oil, Evening Primrose Oil.

AVOID—Heavy meat diet, soft drinks, caffeine, tobacco, heavy starches, all denatured foods. Avoid all sugar products (the downfall of the diabetic). Avoid white flour products. Food containing refined carbohydrates causes the blood sugar to rise quite high during the first two or three hours (diabetes) and then plunges very low at the fourth hour, giving symptoms of low blood sugar (hypoglycemia). The pancreas is wearing out from producing excessive insulin constantly.

DIARRHEA AND DYSENTERY

Diarrhea can be caused from toxic bacteria, colitis, parasites, viruses, chemicals, allergies, antibiotics (destroys friendly bacteria), food poisoning. Diarrhea can be acute or chronic. Diarrhea can be dangerous, especially for babies and young children, because it can lead to loss of body fluids and salts and dehydration. When a child becomes weak with sunken eyes a doctor should be contacted. Diarrhea and dysentery is the way nature takes care of cleansing the body quickly of distress in the body. It could be from parasites or from food poisoning.

Diarrhea is the result of unfriendly bacteria invading the intestinal tract. Poorly cleaned dishes, glasses and silverware can also cause diarrhea. A cutting board can become contaminated if you cut raw meat or chop vegetables or fruit without using a disinfectant.

Some forms of bacteria cause throwing up which helps eliminate contaminated food from the stomach. When contaminated food passes on to the intestinal tract it causes diarrhea. If it enters the blood stream it will cause an infection and if the immune system is low it causes fevers, headaches and other discomforts.

NATURAL THERAPY—Fasting and cleansing the digestive system is the best way to heal and improve diarrhea and dysentery. Enemas will speed up healing using demulcent herbs. Catnip tea is mild and healing for children, as an enema as well as taken internally. Slippery elm will heal. It suppies nutrients and speeds recovery from diarrhea. Use pure water and vegetable juices, especially carrot. Rice water and barley water will heal the digestive system.

FOODS TO HEAL—Bananas contain pectin which will tighten up loose bowels. Carob normalizes the bowels. Unsweetened yogurt. Slippery Elm herb is the best food for diarrhea and dysentery; it will help heal and regulate diarrhea and dysentery.

VITAMINS AND MINERALS—Vitamin A and C, with bioflavonoids will heal the digestive system. B-complex vitamins are lost during diarrhea. Vitamin E for calcium assimilation. Vitamin E protects the cells and veins. Multi-minerals are necessary (lost during diarrhea), extra calcium, potassium (is lost during diarrhea), and zinc. The electrolytes are especially lost during diarrhea.

HERBAL COMBINATIONS—Blood Purifier, Colitis, Digestion, Lower Bowels, Nerves, and Potassium.

SINGLE HERBS—Key herbs: Capsicum (kills germs), Comfrey (soothes and heals irritated mucus membranes), Chamomile Tea (soothing on nerves), Garlic (kills bacteria, parasites and worms), Gentian (heals the digestive system), Ginger (stops cramps), Golden Seal (the greatest healer of the digestive system, kills parasites that can cause diarrhea). Kelp (replaces minerals lost in diarrhea), Pau D'Arco (kills bacteria), Raspberry tea (heals and soothes), Slippery Elm (very healing and soothing), White Oak Bark (heals). Other herbs to help: Alfalfa, Bayberry, Dandelion, Hawthorn, Licorice, Lobelia, Myrrh, Oatstraw (supplies minerals), Red Clover, Wormwood.

SUPPLEMENTS—Acidophilus (replaces bacteria lost in diarrhea), Charcoal Tablets (absorbs toxins and gases), Blackberry Juice (unsweetened), Chlorophyll, Glucomannan, Evening Primrose Oil.

Carob powder is handy to have in controlling diarrhea.

AVOID—Stop eating heavy foods, to give the digestive system a rest and help the body heal itself. Meat is hard on digestion. Avoid sugar products: they irritate the digestive system. Antibiotics destroy friendly bacteria.

DIVERTICULITIS

Diverticulitis is a very common bowel disease. It strikes nearly seventy percent of people past the age of seventy. It usually begins with persistent constipation, which can alternate with diarrhea. It can cause nausea, vomiting, abdominal swelling, cramps and pain. It can even bring a flu-like feeling of chills and fever. Complications may develop causing problems in the bladder, small intestine and uterus. Hemorrhaging and rectal bleeding can occur.

Diverticula are small, pouch-like areas in the large colon. Food enters in the pockets of the large colon and causes infections and toxic material to accumulate. Constipation and a low fiber diet is the main cause of this problem. Straining from hard stools causes pockets in the colon to form, where toxins accumulate. This is another form of autointoxication.

Symptoms are similar to appendicitis except on the left-hand side. There is tenderness, cramping and fever. Chronic diverticulitis can cause irregular bowels, constipation and some pain.

NATURAL THERAPY—The Medical field prescribes a low-residue, soft diet for people with these conditions. But today it is pretty well established that this diet is what created the disease in the first place. A high-fiber diet from whole grains, fruit and vegetables is essential. The first therapy is using demulcent herbs to speed the healing and lower bowel therapy to clean and build up the lower bowels. Blood Purifiers are necessary to clean the organs.

FOODS TO HEAL—Cooked grains: millet, buckwheat, oats (whole), wheat, yellow corn meal, barley. Cooked in a thermos overnight to retain all the enzymes for digestion. Wheatgrass juice speeds healing. Carrot, celery and beet juice. Steamed vegetables blended for easy digestion and assimilation, until healing takes place.

VITAMINS AND MINERALS—Vitamin A (heals and protects the mucus membranes), C (heals and protects immune system), B complex (Improves tone of intestinal tract, builds blood), Vitamin K (Deficiency can cause intestinal disorders). All minerals are needed (liquid for easy assimilation), extra calcium, magnesium, chromium, silicon and zinc.

HERBAL COMBINATIONS—Bone (rich in minerals), Comfrey and Pepsin (comfrey heals and pepsin dissolves toxins), Colitis, Digestion, Lower Bowels, Ulcers.

SINGLE HERBS—Key herbs: Aloe Vera (heals), Alfalfa (rich in minerals as well as K), Comfrey, Fenugreek (cleans and heals colon), Garlic (antibiotic), Glucomannan (cleans colon), Hops (relaxing to colon), Kelp (provides minerals), Marshmallow (healing), Papaya, Psyllium (food for the colon), Slippery Elm (soothes and heals colon). Red Clover Tea. Other beneficial herbs: Dandelion, Lobelia, Myrrh, Pau D'Arco, Scullcap, Yellow Dock.

SUPPLEMENTS—Acidophilus (milk free), Liquid Chlorophyll, Aloe Vera Juice, Bentonite, Fish Oil Lipids, Salmon Oil. Fiber supplements, high fiber cookie.

AVOID—Meat (hard to digest), dairy products, low fiber foods, White sugar and flour products (lack fiber and nourishment).

EAR PROBLEMS

Earaches are very common in childhood. Otitis media is a common childhood infection. Autointoxication is the cause of most ear infections. The blood is poisoned through absorption of toxic material from the intestinal canal. A child may be born with a weakened system and toxins, or they can acquire toxins with a diet of milk products or eating a baby cereal before its teeth develop to provide the enzyme for digestion of grains. Bacteria develops in the ears because of the accumulation of toxins.

A lot of antibiotics are prescribed each year for ear infections. Cases of children with chronic middle ear diseases have increased since the advent of antibiotics. Antibiotics can even cause fluid retention in the ear and prevent healing. A blockage of the eustachian tube is the most common cause of infection. Mucus or inflammation produced when a cold develops, from respiratory infections, allergies, or childhood diseases such as measles, chickenpox, and strep throat can block the small eustachian tube. A child's eustachian tube is shorter than an adult's and can get plugged easily.

Dr. Robert Mendelsohn said that hearing loss is very rare with ear infections. He says that doctors have reinforced our fears. Parents become concerned because of the pain children suffer. The pain is usually caused by pressure that develops when infections interfere with the drainage of the ear through the eustachian tubes.

Foreign objects in the ear and nose are common causes of earaches. They may cause pain or lead to infections, which cause pain. Small children often put things in the nose and ears. I worked for an ear, eyes and nose specialist, and many children were brought in for removal of beans, pieces of paper, cotton balls, jelly beans, pieces of cereal or even safety pins or paper clips.

NATURAL THERAPY—Blood Purification, enemas or lower bowel cleansing will speed the healing. A cleansing diet using citrus juices with liquid or powdered vitamin C will heal as well as clean up infections. Mullein oil in the ears will help with the pain. Garl : and olive oil will heal the infection. Lobelia drops help to ease the pain. If the ear drum is broken, don't put anything in the ear until a doctor has cleaned it out. Applying a warm towel soaked in catnip or chamomile tea will ease the pain. You can alternate the warm towel with a cold towel (not ice) to stimulate circulation which will speed healing. Earaches usually clear up within three to five days by themselves.

Soak the feet in hot water with added tablespoon of mustard or ginger. Roast a lemon in the oven and put a few drops of the juice in the ear (very healing).

FOODS TO HEAL—Freshly juiced citrus fruits, tree ripened if possible. Carrot juice (high in vitamins A and calcium). Vegetable juices and vegetable broths made with celery, potato skins, parsley, and any root and green leafy vegetables.

VITAMINS AND MINERALS—Vitamin A, E or cod liver oil for children (helps control infections), Vitamin C along with calcium helps in healing and preventing infections. B-complex vitamins are healing. Multi-mineral for healing, with extra silicon, selenium and zinc.

HERBAL COMBINATIONS—Blood Purifiers, Lower Bowel Cleansers, Bone combinations.

SINGLE HERBS—Key herbs: Echinacea (natural antibiotic), Fenugreek (loosens mucus), Garlic (natural antibiotic), Ginger (settles stomach), Golden Seal (heals), Hops (relaxes), Lobelia (cleans stomach), Red Clover (cleans blood), Scullcap, Valerian, Yellow Dock. Other beneficial herbs: Aloe Vera, Bayberry, Bilberry, Black Walnut, Burdock, Capsicum, Chaparral, Comfrey, Gotu Kola, Grapevine, Kelp, Lady's Slipper, Oatstraw, Passion Flower, Wood Betony.

SUPPLEMENTS—Liquid Chlorophyll, Acidophilus, Green Drinks, Lemon juice in warm water with pure maple syrup. Herbal teas: Chamomile, Alfalfa-mint, Red Raspberry. Essential Fatty Acids are very healing and essential for children as well as adults. Salmon Oil, Evening Primrose Oil or grind flaxseed to a fine powder and mix with juice or water. (They act more like vitamins in the body.)

AVOID—Milk products. They are mucus forming and increase toxin accumulation. Avoid sugar and white flour products. Avoid a heavy meat diet; use more grains, beans, seeds and nut milk.

ENDOMETRIOSIS

Endometriosis is a rather common disease in our present age. It is estimated that 40 to 60 percent of women who undergo hysterectomies have endometriosis. It is an outgrowth of the uterine lining into the pelvic cavity. It can cause irregular bleeding, pain during intercourse and menstruation, severe pelvic pain and even infertility.

This condition was discovered in 1899 and described in medical journals. In 1920 Dr. J. A. Sampson described the ever increasing disease as very serious. Dr. Sampson found clumps of brown, sticky tissue and old, clotted blood adhering in unusual places: ovaries, rectal ligaments, intestines, and fallopian tubes. (Infertility is increasing at a very high rate). In severe cases, the abdominal organs were glued together and twisted out of place by the contortions of the unusual and strange tissue. Then he discovered that the sticky, clotted tissue was the same as that which lined the normal uterus. It also reacted to the hormonal cycle the same way as the uterine tissue, proliferating when stimulated by estrogen, which would actually bleed during menstruation.

The reason it is hard to diagnosis is it can appear and disappear according to the hormonal profile of the woman. It is not fully understood how the tissue escapes from the uterus in the first place. One theory is that the excess uterine lining is forced upward and out through the fallopian tubes by heavy menstrual contractions. Another theory is that endometrial tissue develops from simple, undifferentiated epithelial cells in the abdomen,like what essentially happens in the female fetus during early pregnancy.

Now physicians realize that endometriosis can probably arise from both of these theories: retrograde menstruation and inappropriate epithelial cell proliferation. Doctors feel that it also stems from other causes not yet discovered. They feel it can also be triggered by episiotomies, IUD'S, cauterization of the cervix and even laparoscopy.

I believe the reason we are seeing more of this disease is because of the excess estrogen we are getting in beef, chicken, turkeys, and in all dairy products: Milk, butter, cottage cheese, sour cream, cream cheese and whipping cream. I also believe that we would be able to handle excess toxins such as artificial hormones if we kept the colon healthy and regular. What happens is the liver becomes overloaded because the bowels are backed up and toxins enter the blood stream to cause problems in the areas where estrogen is used: in the breasts, uterus, vagina and other related parts.

In 1984 an epidemic of early puberty was reported in both males and females all across Puerto Rico. Enlarged breasts in pre-teen children was also reported by health authorities in parts of the continental United States.

Dr. Saenz de Rodriguez in Puerto Rico had seen many cases of premature puberty for several years. She became convinced that the children were being contaminated with estrogen, where four and five-year old girls were suffering from enlarged breasts and ovarian cysts. Milk products , beef and poultry were found to be the problem. The doctor said "we are supposed `to mind our manners' and not question the effects that drugs have upon the population, or your colleagues call you a trouble-maker."

She went on to say, "Much of what we consider healthful growth in our youngsters could be similar to the fattening process the ranchers now use for their cattle. We should not, however, underestimate the time-bomb that is present in those skyrocketing sales figures for fried chicken and hamburgers among young people."

NATURAL THERAPY—Blood Purification and Lower Bowel Therapy will clean and purify the body of excess estrogen and other toxins. Change to a diet using fresh juices from vegetables and fruits. Fruits are cleansing and vegetables are builders with their high mineral content. Instead of a high-meat diet change to brown rice, grains, beans,lentils, peas, and all natural food.

Exercise is very beneficial to prevent adhesions from adhering to the walls of the uterus and other organs. It also helps to normalize hormone levels by metabolizing fat. Activity such as aerobic, stimulates the release of endorphins which are natural opiates that produce a sense of well-being and protect against pain.

FOODS TO HEAL—Vegetables, steamed and fresh. Fresh salads using leaf lettuce, cabbage, carrots, broccoli, and all vegetables. Use olive oil and lemon juice for dressing with garlic, onions, parsley, and vegetable seasonings. Use brown rice, millet, buckwheat, and all whole grains. Thermos cooking will retain the enzymes and B-complex vitamins. Be sure and drink the liquid used to thermos cook. It is rich in enzymes for digestion. Seeds such as sunflower and sesame, almonds and almond milk.

Some women when eliminating sugar, alcohol, caffeine drinks, chocolate and refined foods, while adding B-complex, may at first experience a worsening of symptoms. It is because the ovaries are responding to good nutrition and speed up estrogen production. But with a good diet and clean bowels the liver is able to eliminate the excess estrogen.

VITAMINS AND MINERALS—Vitamins A and E help heal and protect against scar tissue, and aid in hormone imbalance. Vitamin C and bioflavonoids are essential in healing and cleansing the body. B-complex vitamins are very important. They are lost every day, and stress rapidly depletes the body of these vitamins. Extra B6 with magnesium will reduce symptoms of estrogen overload. Remember the liver is the site of eliminating excess estrogen, and it cannot do it without adequate B vitamins.

Multi-minerals are very important. Especially iron (found in Yellow Dock), iodine (found in kelp), and calcium and magnesium found in calcium herbal formulas. Selenium, zinc and silicon are important.

HERBAL COMBINATIONS—Blood Purifiers, Female, Glands, Immune, Lower Bowels, Nerves, and Stress.

SINGLE HERBS—Key Herbs: Black Cohosh, Cramp Bark, Damiana, Dong Quai, False Unicorn, Gentian, Ginseng, Gotu Kola, Kelp, Licorice, Sarsaparilla, Saw Palmetto, Squaw Vine and Wild Yam. Other important herbs: Alfalfa, Black Walnut, Burdock (cleans blood), Capsicum (circulation to speed healing), Chaparral (cleans blood and liver), Dandelion (cleans liver), Garlic, Ginger, Golden Seal (clears infections), Hops, Ho Shou-Wu, Hawthorn, Irish Moss, Lobelia, Mistletoe, Myrrh, Red Clover (blood cleanser), Scullcap (cleans veins and restores nerves), Watercress, Wood Betony, Wormwood, Yellow Dock.

SUPPLEMENTS—Free form Amino Acids; Essential Fatty Acids in Salmon and fish liver oils. Lecithin, Spirulina, Pancreatic enzymes and Hydrochloric acid if needed. Chlorophyll cleans the blood.

AVOID—All products that have hormones added: Meat, poultry, milk, cheese, cottage cheese, butter, sour cream, whipping cream. Avoid sugar, it depletes the body of needed B-complex vitamins and calcium. Avoid estrogen therapies, if possible. Caffeine and chocolate aggravate female problems.

ENVIRONMENTAL POISONING

Environmental toxins are a real health problem. They are in our water, food and air. Herbicide and pesticide residues are everywhere. We are constantly being exposed, and residue samples are found in the blood and urine of both urban and rural areas. These poisons are capable of causing mutations and cancer. It has also been found in mothers' milk. Lindane (bug bombs) used in home gardens, and on farms for treating seeds and hardwood lumber as well as in animal shampoos, flea collars, shelf paper and floor wax. It can cause cancer, is toxic to a growing fetus, damaging to the reproductive organs, toxic to fish, and children are very susceptible.

We are threatened with electromagnetic radiation which has been linked to leukemia. We have food additives, preservatives, artificial coloring, sprays on our fruits to ripen them artificially, and colors to enhance their selling ability. We are bombarded with all kinds of pollution.

Radiation poisoning suppresses an already weakened immune system. When you undergo radiation therapy you may experience radiation burns and scarring, fatigue and puts a strain on the immune system. Radiation destroys many nutrients in the body.

Supplements are vital to improve immune function and protect the system of diseases.

NATURAL THERAPY—Keep the immune system strong and the liver clean in order to eliminate the toxins we breathe and eat. Blood, liver and lower bowels need to be kept clean and in good working order. We need to demand food that is free from additives and other chemicals.

FOODS TO HEAL—Green leafy vegetables, whole grains, beans, high fiber foods, broccoli, cabbage, kale, carrots, spinach, green peppers.

VITAMINS AND MINERALS—Vitamin A (helps detoxify toxins as well as protect the immune system), B-complex (protects the cells) with extra B5, B6, and B12 to protect against stress, C with bioflavonoids (heals and protects the immune system). Vitamin E (protects against free radicals, heals and protects against radiation burns), Minerals are essential. They act as chelating agents to metals and other toxins. Calcium helps take lead out of the body; selenium protects the immune system along with zinc. Silicon helps protect the bones.

HERBAL COMBINATIONS—Blood Purifiers, Chelating, Bone (rich in minerals), Immune formulas, Nerve and Stress Formulas. Lower Bowel formulas help to eliminate toxins the liver filters.

SINGLE HERBS—Alfalfa, Aloe Vera (heals and protects against burns), Burdock (purifies blood and eliminates toxins), Capsicum (increases circulation for rapid healing), Chaparral (cleans blood and eliminates poisons), Comfrey (healing), Echinacea (cleans blood and lymphatic system), Garlic (natural antibiotic), Ginkgo (healing and promotes brain function), Golden Seal (healing for mucus membranes), Juniper Berries, Kelp (supplies minerals to eliminate poisons), Lobelia, Mullein, Parsley, Pau D'Arco (cleans blood and protects liver), Red Clover (blood cleanser), Sarsaparilla, Suma, Watercress, Yellow Dock.

SUPPLEMENTS—Acidophilus, Liquid Chlorophyll, Bee Pollen, Blue-green Algae, Wheat grass juice, Barley green drinks, Germanium, CoQ10, Amino Acids (L-carnitine, glutathione, L-Methionine, L-Cysteine).

AVOID—Avoid all food additives. Frozen food contains a lot of preservatives. Second-hand tobacco smoke will harm the lungs.

Children are very susceptible to smoke. Avoid sugar and all white flour products. Meat has antibiotics and hormones and fried foods will weaken the immune system.

EPILEPSY

In *The Ultimate Healing System* by Donald LePore, N.D., he states, "We believe that epilepsy is not a disease, but is actually nature's way of getting rid of the deteriorating matter on the brain. The epileptic seizure is like an electrical storm; this is nature's way of giving an electrical charge to correct the malfunction of the brain which sometimes is scar tissue in the area."

The actual epileptic seizure is due to a sudden, abnormal and excessive electrical discharge within the brain. In primary epilepsy the basic cause is unknown; there is usually a genetic predisposition. Secondary epilepsy can be from a head injury, bacterial meningitis and malaria; it is often associated with cerebral palsy, mental retardation, brain tumors and cysts and hydrocephalus.

There are drugs that can cause epilepsy or aggravate existing epileptic disorders:Amphetamines, antihistamine, chloroquine, cimetidine, cycloserine, monoamine oxidase inhibitors, oral contraceptives, phenothiazines, tricyclic antidepressants.

Dilantin is the most widely prescribed medication for epilepsy. It works on the motor cortex to stop the spread of seizure activity. There are precautions when using this drug: it can cause mental confusion, dizziness, vomiting and constipation.

NATURAL THERAPY—Blood Purification and Lower Bowel Cleansing. Prevent toxins from entering the blood, by keeping the bowels moving every day. A high fiber diet with wholesome food will help nourish the brain and nervous system. The brain is very sensitive to toxins from the blood.

FOODS TO HEAL—Fresh fruit and juices, raw and steamed vegetables, whole grains, sprouts from seeds and grains, green drinks, and eat as much raw food to nourish the brain and nerves. Thermos cooking of grains helps to retain enzymes, and vitamins and minerals essential for brain nourishment. Fresh green salads should be eaten every day.

VITAMINS AND MINERALS—B-complex vitamins, especially Folic acid and B12, which are quickly destroyed when taking dilantin or phenobarbital. All B vitamins are important. Vitamins A, C and E provide protection to the immune system. Niacin, choline (is needed to form acetylcholine, a major neurotransmitter that can improve memory). Minerals are essential for brain health. Sodium deficiency can cause brain malfunction. Calcium and magnesium feed and nourish the brain and nervous system. Selenium, silicon and zinc help to nourish the gland and brain. Manganese deficiency is seen in epileptics. B6 helps to prevent convulsions.

HERBAL COMBINATIONS—Blood cleanser, digestion, Glands, Nerve, Lower Bowels. Herbs are very beneficial to the nervous system and brain function.

SINGLE HERBS—Key herbs: Black Walnut (parasites can cause epilepsy), Burdock (cleans blood), Capsicum, Echinacea (cleans glands), Garlic, Ginkgo (stimulates brain), Gotu Kola (food for the brain), Hawthorn, Hops (nerves), Lady's Slipper (strengthens brain function), Lobelia, Passion Flower, Pau D'Arco (cleans blood and liver), Red Clover, Scullcap (brain relaxer), Valerian. Other important herbs: Alfalfa, Black Cohosh, Dandelion, Gentian, Ginger, Licorice, Yellow Dock.

SUPPLEMENTS—Acidophilus, Lecithin, Psyllium, Glucomannan, Bee Pollen, Spirulina, Senna tea, Rice Bran Syrup. Hydrochloric Acid (aids in digestion and removal of toxic material that interferes with brain function). Taurine, Tryptophan and Glutamine, detoxifies ammonia from the brain. All Amino Acids are essential for brain health. Chlorophyll cleans the blood.

AVOID—Avoid all denatured food. Sugar is detrimental to the body as well as the brain. White flour lacks essential minerals and is lacking in fiber. Tobacco, caffeine and alcohol are very harmful to the brain and nervous system. Avoid fried food: they cause free radicals and destruction to the cells.

EPSTEIN-BARR VIRUS

Epstein-Barr Virus is also called Chronic Fatigue Syndrome and the "Fatigue Disease". It is becoming very widespread and is a common virus that usually remains dormant in most people, but when the immune system is lowered it is one of the diseases that is triggered. It has been around for a long time and causes infectious mononucleosis, the "kissing disease" that often strikes young people. The Epstein-Barr virus causes both diseases, but mononucleosis strikes all at once, hits hard and usually lasts two to four weeks or may linger longer. EBV is chronic and lingers for months and maybe even years.

EBV symptoms are: fatigue that leaves you exhausted, recurrent upper-respiratory tract infections, swollen lymph nodes, memory loss, achy joints and muscles, low-grade fevers, headaches, night sweats, poor concentration, irritability, and serious depression.

In the past, EBVS has been misdiagnosed as a psychosomatic problem. Epstein-Barr Virus depletes the body's natural immunity, leaving it susceptible to a number of illnesses.

NATURAL THERAPY—Blood Purification and Lower Bowel Cleanse. Short fasts to clean the blood, using juices and pure water. Carrot, celery, parsley juices. Green drinks to purify the blood. Bed rest and relaxation therapy will help speed healing.

FOODS TO HEAL—Citrus fruit (rich in vitamin C), Cherries, parsley, green peppers, watercress, kale, broccoli, fresh salads with lots of raw vegetables.

VITAMINS AND MINERALS—Vitamin A (build the immune system), B-complex (with extra folic acid, B12). Vitamin C (with bioflavonoids, to strengthen the immune system and heal). Multi-mineral, healing and essential for the body. Extra selenium, silicon and zinc.

HERBAL COMBINATIONS—Blood Purifier (Red Clover blends), Digestion, Infection (containing herbs and vitamins), Liver (helps to detoxify the toxins), Nerve and stress herbal formulas.

SINGLE HERBS—Key herbs: Echinacea (cleans glands), Garlic (antibiotic), Golden Seal (cleans and heals), Horsetail, Lobelia, Oatstraw, Pau D'Arco (blood cleanser), Red Clover, Saffron (helps to stop aches and pains), Scullcap (helps the nerves). Other beneficial herbs: Aloe Vera, Buchu, Burdock, Capsicum, Comfrey, Cornsilk, Dandelion, Ginger, Hawthorn, Licorice, Myrrh, Parsley, Watercress, Yellow Dock.

SUPPLEMENTS—Bee Pollen, Acidophilus, Evening Primrose oil or Salmon Oil, Garlic Oil, Chlorophyll, Rice Bran Syrup.

AVOID—Sugar depletes calcium and B-vitamins. Caffeine drinks lower the immune system and deplete potassium and other minerals from the body. Avoid fried foods, high fat foods, white sugar products. Avoid antibiotics—they will not help in viruses.

EYE PROBLEMS

Eyesight is a precious gift. At least eighty percent of the decisions we make each day are based on information we receive through using our vision. Yet more than ten million people in the United States suffer severe vision disability. The medical profession gives them no hope. The drugs they prescribe and the surgery they perform or lenses offer them no relief.

Retinitis pigmentosa (an inherited genetic eye disease) is when the retina's nerve elements causes progressive atrophy, where clumping of pigment and finally atrophy of the optic disks. Night blindness is one of the first signs. Other diseases of the eyes, other than eye infections, are senile macular degeneration, diabetic retinopathy, optic nerve atrophy and cataracts. All of these will increase blindness by 160 percent in the next 40 years.

In the United States many eye specialists feel that clogged up blood vessels and junk food are big contributors to blindness. The eye, along with the brain, requires more nutrition and circulation than any other single body organ.

Millions of electric waves travel from the optic nerve to the brain, which is constantly draining and drawing fuel from the nutrition our bodies supply. Poor nutrition clogs up tiny arteries, veins, and capillaries that support the visual system. The gradual clogging, which had been traced to poor nutrition, can result in eventual blindness.

Common drugs have an adverse effect on the eyes. Sedative drugs such as tranquilizers and sleeping pills destroy the electrochemical balance which interferes with nerve transmission by putting "foreign energies" as well as preventing vital nutrients from entering the eyes.

Air pollution, especially tobacco smoke, can cause burning, dry, itchy, irritated and blood shot eyes. Through iridology the eyes can help determine weaknesses in other parts of the body. In fact eye problems are often an early indication of diseases in the body. Dark circles under the eyes are a sign of allergies, watery and red eyes are a sign of a cold coming on; bulging eyes can indicate a thyroid problem. Yellowing of the eyes are an indication of hepatitis, liver problems or gall bladder problems. An eye specialist can see signs of high blood pressure and diabetes in patients when doing a regular eye examination.

NATURAL THERAPY—Good nutrition is vital to maintain good eyesight and prevention is always better than the cure. Blood purification, and Lower bowel cleansing are essential.

Natural herbal eyewash will cleanse and stimulate circulation to the eye tissues. Use often to prevent clogging up of the tiny capillaries and veins. The eyes absorb toxins from the lower bowel, what we call autointoxication, a self poisoning. A liver cleanse and bowel cleanse with enemas, colonics or using lower bowel cleansers will improve eyesight and other problems. It takes patience and perseverance.

Foot reflexology has a direct stimulation effect on the eyes and brain. It will help promote circulation in the eye area.

FOODS TO HEAL—Whole grain (thermos cooking to retain the enzymes), millet, buckwheat, whole oats, wheat, barley, and all whole grains, brown rice, yellow corn meal, beans of all kinds. Green leafy vegetables, whole nuts and seeds, and a lot of raw and steamed vegetables. Avocados are high in vitamin A and Protein. Carrots and raw carrot juice are rich in vitamin A and Calcium.

VITAMINS AND MINERALS—Vitamin A (helps prevent night blindness), protects the eyes from irritations, and protects from dry eyes. B-complex vitamins (helps prevent eye sensitivity and itching) extra B2; deficiency shows in people with itching, eye irritation, and poor adaptability to light changes. Niacin clears out the fatty deposits from the tiny blood vessel, and improves blood flow, B6 will lower the ocular pressure. Inositol is necessary for healthy eye membranes. Vitamin C with bioflavonoids protects against the formation of cataracts, it is abundantly found in the lens of the eyes. Vitamin C and E protects against cellular deterioration caused by smoke, junk food and air pollution. They both carry oxygen to the cells. Prolonged mineral deficiency can result in squinting, distorted visual perception, vertigo, fatigue and headaches and painful eyes. Zinc is necessary for the transformation of vitamin A. Chromium and zinc protect against cataracts. Calcium is important to the connective tissues of the eyes. Deficiency results in a softening of the outer shell of the eyeball.

HERBAL COMBINATIONS—Blood Purifiers, Digestion, Eye Formulas, Infection (when infected, Lower Bowels and Stress.

SINGLE HERBS—Key herbs: Bilberry (strengthens eyes), Capsicum (cleans capillaries), Eyebright (improves eyes), Golden Seal (cleans veins), Hops, Lobelia, Passion Flower (improves nerves), Scullcap, Valerian. Other beneficial herbs: Aloe Vera, Bayberry, Black Cohosh, Black Walnut, Burdock, Chaparral, Comfrey, Echinacea, Fenugreek, Garlic, Ginger, Ginseng, Gotu Kola, Grapevine, Hawthorn, Myrrh, Oatstraw, Red Clover, White Oak and Yellow Dock.

SUPPLEMENTS—Evening Primrose Oil, Salmon Oil, Chlorophyll, Lecithin. Taurine, an amino acid protects tissues under stress. Cod Liver Oil. Free Form Amino Acids, essential for eye health.

AVOID—Caffeine (too much), has an adverse effect on the ability of the eyes to focus for reading or other close work. Sugar depletes calcium and B Vitamins that are essential for eye health. Cigarette smoke is very harmful on the eyes. Tinted eyeglass prevents light from entering the eyes.

FATIGUE

   Lack of energy affects your vitality, emotions and personal relationships. In fact it will affect your whole life, as well as your happiness . Fatigue is a very serious symptom that needs to be addressed. You wake up in the morning tired and go to bed tired. It is a hopeless feeling that is hard to shake. Fatigue can stem from a multitude of conditions. Physicians and health practitioners are seeing a tiredness in patients that have no obvious cause. This fatigue is a symptom and a warning of the body telling you to find the cause. It can be emotional, mental, spiritual, psychological and physical.

   Common causes of fatigue are: anemia, allergies, autointoxication, candida, Epstein-Barr virus, hypoglycemia, hypothyroidism, toxic metal poisoning, physical stress, lack of nutrients.

   Fatigue or exhaustion cannot usually be dealt with by additional rest. There has to be a change in diet, thinking and a holistic approach to this symptom. Negative thinking has a very profound detrimental effect on the body. Any type of stress can cause complete exhaustion. A person with a strong constitution can probably endure more stress than someone with a weak constitution, but it will eventually catch up with them. Another sign of fatigue is that a person cannot cope with situations the way they used to.

Constant frustration and anger for no apparent reason is another sign of exhaustion and fatigue. Loss of sexual desire is another sign of fatigue. I believe this is one reason people turn to drugs and stimulants is to try and recapture the energy they once had. I believe the underlying cause is lack of nutrients being assimilated in the body. Autointoxication and digestive problems are the main cause.

NATURAL THERAPY—Fatigue is a symptom of a toxic body not assimilating nutrients necessary for energy. The blood needs to be purified with Blood Purifiers. The colon needs to be cleaned with Lower Bowel Cleaners, enemas, or colonics. With the proper diet and cleansing program the body will gradually gain strength and energy. It may take months or years, but patience and a positive attitude will speed the healing.

Exercise and obtain fresh air once you start gaining strength. The cells needs oxygen. Deep breathing will also bring energy to the cells.

Stimulation through Chiropractic treatments restores balance to the brain and nervous system. The brain has the knowledge to correct problems that exist in different areas of the body. Along with nutrition, health can be restored.

FOODS TO HEAL—Fresh vegetables and steamed vegetables (contain minerals to prevent fatigue), Fresh fruit and juices (cleansing and healing), whole grains, either slow or thermos cooking to retain nutrients (B-complex vitamins , enzymes and minerals), seeds (sesame, sunflower, pumpkin), nuts (almonds, pecans, filberts, and cashews).

VITAMINS AND MINERALS—Multi-vitamin supplement (yeast free), with extra B6, B12. Pantothenic Acid (promotes energy). Vitamin C with bioflavonoids. Vitamin E, to get oxygen to the cells. Multi-minerals (liquid for assimilation). Extra calcium and magnesium (balance), chromium, iron, potassium, selenium and zinc.

HERBAL COMBINATIONS—Anemia, Blood Purifier, Bone (minerals), Candida, Digestion, Energy, Hypoglycemia, Immune, Lower Bowels.

SINGLE HERBS—Key Herbs: Capsicum, Dong Quai, Ginkgo (strengthens the body), Ginseng (energy booster, helps restore energy reserves by increasing carbohydrate metabolism and glycogen storage), Gotu Kola (food for the brain), Hawthorn, Ho Shou-Wu (tonic for the glands), Licorice (provides energy and balances hormones), Red Clover (cleans blood for clearer thinking), Schizandra (improves oxygen utilization and restores energy reserve), Suma (stimulates brain function). Other beneficial herbs: Alfalfa, Black Cohosh, Burdock, Chaparral, Dandelion, Garlic, Ginger, Gentian (heals digestive system), Golden Seal, Hops (heals the nerves), Lobelia, Mistletoe, Myrrh, Scullcap (strengthens the brain and nerves), St. Johnswort, Valerian, Wood Betony, Wormwood, Yellow Dock.

SUPPLEMENTS—Acidophilus, Bee Pollen, Chlorophyll, Herbal teas (oatstraw, red raspberry,), Evening Primrose Oil, Salmon Oil. Co Q10, Germanium. Lecithin (quick energy to the brain).

AVOID-All stimulants deplete the body of needed energy. Alcohol, tobacco, caffeine. Chocolate, soft drinks, candy and any sugar foods are stimulating to an already weakened body. Meat and processed food robs the body of vital nutrients.

FIBROCYSTIC DISEASE
(female)

Fibrocystic breast disease involves over fifty percent of adult females in the United States. This is a benign lump condition which only rarely turns cancerous. The anguish it causes to many women is worth learning about. In the past it has been described as a hormonal upset and is still regarded as such to many physicians. In a way it is a hormonal imbalance. Many health nutritionist believe that the problem stems from too much "unfavorable" estrogen, called estradiol, a type of estrogen that the liver cannot filter because of congestion in the colon. This bad estrogen is responsible for proliferating tissue, where it travels to the primary estrogen receptors of the body (especially in the breasts and uterus), which causes cysts and growths. Estradiol as well as other toxins back up into the blood stream and enter the breasts, brain or other parts of the body to cause lumps, congestion or other diseases in the system. When the liver is congested, it cannot filter harmful substances such as caffeine, found in coffee, tea, cola and chocolate.

NATURAL THERAPY—A Liver and Lower Bowel cleanse is essential. A high fiber diet is beneficial. Changing the dietary habits is necessary for a healthy liver to filter toxins that cause cysts, lumps and cancerous growths. Blood Purification therapy will help the healing process. Avoid meat; it contains hormones (estrogen). Antibiotics increase the chances of breast lumps. The bowels must be kept active.

FOODS TO HEAL—Almonds, sesame and sunflower seeds, raw fruits and green leafy vegetables and sprouts. High fiber diet using whole grains and vegetables will help prevent growths. Potassium foods (cysts and growths cannot live in a high potassium environment): Dulse, Kelp, Irish moss, Lima beans, rice bran, whole grains, bananas, white and pinto beans, mung beans (sprouted), dried peas, apricots, pistachio nuts, peach (dried), lentils, chickpeas, parsley, prunes.

Fresh lemon juice in warm water will help cleanse the liver. Green drinks, such as wheat grass juice, will clean the blood and liver.

VITAMINS AND MINERALS—Vitamin A protects the body from cancer causing toxins. A deficiency contributes to growths. B-complex, especially pantothenic acid, niacin, and riboflavin protects against cysts and growths. The liver cannot eliminate estradiol without B vitamins, especially choline and inositol. B6 is necessary to manufacture progesterone, an estrogen antagonist. B15 increases the body's resistance to oxygen deficiency (oxygen deficiency causes cancer and tumors to invade the cells). B vitamins are leached from the liver if too much sugar, processed starches and alcohol are present.

Vitamin C (neutralizes the damaging effect of carcinogenic material in food), Vitamin E, powerful antioxidant helps prevent fat oxidation and formation of free radicals, which cause breast cancer.

A multi-mineral is vital for a healthy body. Calcium and magnesium (found in herbs such as Horsetail) are excellent in balancing minerals. Iodine (found in Kelp), and Zinc enhances the body's ability to make use of essential fatty acids. Selenium protects the body against toxins.

HERBAL COMBINATIONS—Blood Purifiers, Digestion, Glands, Immune, Lower Bowels, Nerve, Potassium.

SINGLE HERBS—Key herbs: Burdock, Chaparral, Dandelion (cleans liver), Echinacea (cleans glands), Garlic, Golden Seal, Kelp, Milk Thistle, Pau D'Arco (protects liver from toxins), Red Clover (drink Red Clover blend teas), Yellow Dock.

SUPPLEMENTS—Acidophilus (friendly bacteria), Liquid Chlorophyll, Lecithin, Evening Primrose Oil, Salmon Oil, or Flax seeds contain essential fatty acids.

AVOID—Sugar, leaches B vitamins, Reduce fat intake—excess fat causes chronic diseases. Eliminate coffee, chocolate, tea and caffeine soft drinks; they contains chemicals under the name of methylxanthines. Avoid alcohol and drugs: they destroy vitamins and minerals and promote fibrous growths and cysts. White flour products have no nutritional value and congest the liver and colon.

FOOD POISONING

Food poisoning can be very serious if it isn't taken care of properly. Nature usually takes over and causes diarrhea and vomiting to rid the body of toxins. Symptoms of food poisoning include diarrhea, nausea, vomiting and cramps lasting from a few hours to a few days. It usually lasts twenty-four hours. When it lasts longer it is usually thought to be the flu.

The body has a natural way of dealing with poisons and toxins, worms, and parasites that enter our bodies. It naturally produces hydrochloric acid, which kills and destroys toxins and is a protection for the digestive system. But, because of the typical American diet, (which is very high in sugar, white flour products, meat and fried oil) it destroys the body's ability to produce this acid. Therefore, toxins can enter and cause us much distress.

There are many kinds of food poisoning: Botulism, Salmonella, Staphylococcus aureus, Clostridium botulinum (called Cafeteria botulinum), and Giardiasis (associated with contaminated water).

Care must be taken in preparing food; it should not be left out of the refrigerator. If you use eggs, be very careful. They are susceptible to Salmonella bacteria. Left out potato salad can cause problems. Canned food with bulging tops should never be used. Just use common sense when preparing and eating food and you can avoid food poisoning. Salmonella poisoning can be contracted from chicken, eggs, beef and pork products. Handling meat and poorly cooked meat can cause this poison to thrive. Use Clorox water after handling raw meat to protect against salmonella.

NATURAL THERAPY—Keep the blood clean and pure with blood purifier herbs. Using herbs that kill bacteria (Golden Seal, Garlic) will help keep the intestinal tract clean. Change to a natural diet, which will help prevent germs and bacteria from forming. Bacteria, germs and toxins will not live in a clean body.

FOODS TO HEAL—Citrus juices diluted with pure water. Vegetable potassium broths (potato peelings, onions, garlic, parsley, celery as well as other vegetables, strain and drink the broth). Herbal teas soothe the stomach. After vomiting use mint teas which will calm the stomach (peppermint, spearmint, catnip and chamomile, and alfalfa-mint tea are healing).

Nature usually prevents you from being hungry, but if you are, don't eat; it will only stop the cleansing and drive the toxins further into the system where it will later cause chronic disease.

VITAMINS AND MINERALS—Vitamin A (emulsion, enters system faster), Liquid vitamin C, with bioflavonoids (will help detoxify and strengthen the body). Multi-minerals (depleted quickly when vomiting especially potassium. (Herbal mineral formula is best.)

HERBAL COMBINATIONS—Blood Purifiers, Digestion, Colds and Flu, Lower Bowels, Nerves, Stress.

SINGLE HERBS—Key herbs: Catnip (calms the stomach), Garlic (natural antibiotic), Gentian (healing for the digestive system), Ginger (calming for upset stomach), Golden Seal (heals the digestive system), Kelp (cleans and provides minerals), Red Clover. Other important herbs: Alfalfa, Aloe Vera (cleansing and healing), Bayberry, Black Walnut (kills worms and parasites), Buckthorn, Burdock, Capsicum, Cascara Sagrada, Chaparral, Dandelion, Echinacea, Ginseng, Hawthorn, Irish Moss, Licorice, Lobelia (cleans the stomach), Myrrh, Psyllium, Watercress, Yarrow, Yellow Dock.

SUPPLEMENTS—Free-form Amino acids(enter system quickly for tissue repair), Acidophilus (replace friendly bacteria that is lost with diarrhea and vomiting), Ipecac (induce vomiting), Charcoal (absorbs toxins). Blue-green algae (clean and repairs cells).

AVOID—All sugar products, fried foods, white flour products, meat, cheese, drugs; (will only weaken the body more). Stop eating this is the best thing you can do so the body can heal itself the way nature intended.

FRACTURES

A broken bone can happen to anyone. We need to contact a doctor to make sure the bone will be set properly to prevent poor healing and a crippled limb.

The bones are capable of supporting heavy loads and are a storehouse of calcium and other minerals. They are the seat of the vital red blood cells, which protects the delicate body parts, and the joints that allows us to move about freely. There is a good reason to take care of our bones.

We can prevent sports injuries such as runner's knee, tennis elbow, torn cartilage and ligaments and broken or dislocated bones, as well as heal these injuries faster with a wholesome diet that includes lots of minerals.

Bones, even though they are strong, suffer weakness when injuries, genetic weakness, metabolic disorders, and aging take place. They do not have to be weak if we take care in keeping them strong and healthy. It doesn't matter how old you get—your bones can repair themselves with proper nutrients. Even scoliosis and curvature of the spine can be helped. Bones are comprised of minerals, calcium and phosphorus deposited on a type of protein which is called collagen. Collagen formation requires vitamin C with bioflavonoids for healthy bones and connective tissues.

NATURAL THERAPY—See a doctor for proper healing of bones to take place. Drink vegetable juices (carrot, celery, parsley), and vegetable broths. These, as well as fresh salads, contain a lot of minerals for healing. Herbs also contain a lot of minerals especially good for bone healing.

FOODS TO HEAL—Broccoli, Sprouted Grains, Kale Leaves, Parsley, Carrot juice, Whey Powder, and homemade sauerkraut.

VITAMINS AND MINERALS—Vitamin A is essential for healing (vital for protein assimilation). Vitamin C with bioflavonoids will speed the healing. B-vitamins speed healing. Vitamin D, along with calcium, is necessary for bone repair. Selenium and zinc will also expedite healing. Silicon is the king of bone healers (found in oatstraw and horsetail). Calcium and magnesium are essential for bone healing. (I prefer the herbal calcium formulas.) Potassium and sodium balance will help keep the swelling under control. Trace minerals such as copper, manganese and zinc are important for bone formation.

HERBAL COMBINATIONS—Bone formulas, Digestion, Lower Bowel, Potassium, Nerves (help keep the pain under control).

SINGLE HERBS—Key herbs: Alfalfa (rich in minerals), Aloe Vera (healing and cleansing), Capsicum, Comfrey (promotes bone healing), Dandelion, Garlic, Gentian, Golden Seal (cleans the digestive tract), Hops (helps in pain), Horsetail (repairs bones with rich silicon content), Kelp (rich in minerals), Scullcap (helps relax muscles), Wood Betony (acts as a tranquilizer), Yellow Dock. Other beneficial herbs: Black Cohosh, Burdock, Chaparral, Dong Quai, Ginseng, Gotu Kola, Hawthorn, Lobelia, Mistletoe.

SUPPLEMENTS—Blue-green Algae (increases healing), Liquid Chlorophyll, flaxseed (essential fatty acids), Liquid minerals for faster assimilation. Hydrochloric acid and Pancreatic enzymes for assimilation of minerals.

AVOID—All sugar products (leaches calcium from bones), caffeine, and cola drinks. White flour products (void of B-vitamins and minerals). Chocolate leaches calcium and B-vitamins from bones.

GOUT

The tendency to get gout can be hereditary, which means you can be born with the weakness for this disease. It doesn't mean you have to be plagued by this ailment. Too much uric acid in the blood and tissues causes gout. It crystalizes in the joints and creates swelling and pain from the abrasive action of the uric acid crystals.

Attacks can occur in the night with pain in the joint of the big toe. It is usually swollen, red and tender to the touch. Wrist, ankle or thumb joints may be affected. Gout has been associated with drinking beer, wine and a high meat diet.

NATURAL THERAPY—Blood Purification and Colon Cleanse will help this ailment. Foot Reflexology will help break up the crystals, and blood purifiers (herbal) will help eliminate the crystals out of the body. Foot reflexology may be painful but worth it to get rid of this ailment, which causes pain.

FOODS TO HEAL—Raw vegetable juices (carrot, celery, parsley), green drinks, rich in chlorophyll. Cherry juice (unsweetened). Vegetable broths, using potato peelings, celery with leaves, onions, parsley, and other vegetables, strained and drink the broth, contains potassium and other minerals to dissolve uric acid deposits.

VITAMINS AND MINERALS—Vitamin A (an antioxidant, prevents toxins from accumulating in joints), B-complex vitamins aid in metabolism. Vitamin C with bioflavonoids (they work together, eliminating uric acid from blood). Vitamin E, increases circulation and destroys free radicals (which destroys cells and creates toxins). Multi-minerals (eliminate uric acid and creates healing). Selenium and zinc help in tissue repair and healing bones.

HERBAL COMBINATIONS—Arthritis formulas, Blood Purifiers, Bone, Digestion, Nerve and Pain formulas.

SINGLE HERBS—Alfalfa, Aloe Vera, Brigham Tea, Burdock (blood purifier), Capsicum (helps in circulation), Chaparral (cleans blood and uric acid), Comfrey (healing), Dandelion (cleans liver to filter uric acid), Devil's Claw (cleanses vascular walls, and eliminates toxin from the blood), Dulse (rich in minerals), Garlic, Hydrangea (helps kidneys to eliminate uric acid), Kelp (rich in minerals for cleansing and healing), Parsley, Papaya, Saffron, Red Clover, Watercress, White Willow, Yucca (anti-stress properties).

SUPPLEMENTS—Free-form Amino Acids, Cystine (works with pantothenic acid in gout treatment), Histidine (removes heavy metals and toxins), Phenylalanine (for pain). Distilled water, Green Drinks, CO Q10, Fish Oil Lipids, Salmon Oil, Evening Primrose Oil, Chinese Essential oils and Tea Tree Oil (for external use).

AVOID—All meat (very high in uric acid). White flour and sugar products only increases the ailment. Rich foods such as cakes, pies, ice cream, candy only irritate the problem. Sardines, high salt diet, organ meats, meat gravies and broths will aggravate gout.

GUILLAIN-BARRE SYNDROME

Guillain-Barre syndrome is a disease causing muscle weakness and inflammation of nerve roots. The disease affects the myelin sheath (protects the nerves), of the neuron, which leads to muscle loss and can lead to paralysis.

In 1976 President Gerald Ford authorized a nation wide vaccination program against the swine flu. The project ran into difficulties from the start and was abandoned after the vaccine was found to cause Guillain-Barre syndrome. Flu shots reduce the concentration of some vital enzymes in the liver, which could lead to a build up of drugs, poisons and viruses in the blood stream.

NATURAL THERAPY—Blood Purification and Nervine Therapy are the most effective treatments. This disease damages the nerves, so care must be taken to drink and eat food to repair the myelin sheath. Chiropractic treatments will stimulate circulation to help repair nerves. Foot Reflexology will also repair and heal the nerves.

FOODS TO HEAL—Fresh and steamed vegetables. Sprouted seeds, nuts and grains. Thermos cooking of grains, to retain vitamins, minerals and enzymes.

Fresh vegetable salads. Fresh fruit. High fiber diet using whole oats, oat bran and whole grains such as millet, buckwheat, wheat, barley, rye.

VITAMINS AND MINERALS—Vitamin A (healing for mucus membranes), B-complex (extra B5, Pantothenic acid, and B12 for nerves), C with bioflavonoids for healing and cleansing. Multi-minerals with extra calcium, magnesium, selenium, silicon and zinc.

HERBAL COMBINATIONS—Blood Purifiers, Bone (for calcium and other essential minerals). Digestion, Glands, Nerve, Lower Bowels, Potassium and stress formulas.

SINGLE HERBS—Key herbs: Black Cohosh (tonic for the nerves), Blue Vervain (natural tranquilizer), Catnip (calms stomach and nerves), Chamomile (contains tryptophan with sedative properties), Echinacea (cleans the lymphatics), Gentian (stimulates circulation for healing), Ginkgo (stimulates brain function), Hops (heals nerves), Horsetail, Kelp, Lady's Slipper, Lobelia, Passion Flower, Psyllium, Red Clover, Scullcap (feeds and heals the nerves), Suma, Valerian. Other important herbs: Alfalfa, Aloe Vera, Black Walnut, Buchu, Burdock, Capsicum, Cascara Sagrada, Dandelion, Ginger, Hawthorn, Juniper, Licorice, Parsley, Uva Ursi, Yellow Dock.

SUPPLEMENTS—Evening Primrose Oil, Salmon Oil, Lecithin (strengthens the myelin sheath). Germanium, CO Q10.

AVOID—Sugar products deplete essential vitamins and minerals that heal the nerves). Avoid fried foods (creates free radicals that will destroy cells). Avoid refined foods, canned foods and any foods with additives and preservatives. Monosodium glutamate is harmful to the nerves.

HAIR HEALTH

Beautiful hair adds to a persons attractiveness but it also has practical purposes. It conserves body heat and protects the scalp and it plays a role in the sensory system. The hair follicles, which are at the root of each hair shaft, are surrounded by sensory nerves that react whenever the hair shaft is touched or brushed.

The hair shaft is the part that grows above the skins surface. This part of the hair is alive. Hair is not dead tissue but is growing continuously. It is alive and is affected by hormones, enzymes, blood, perspiration, environment and genetics. The use of dyes, chemicals, permanents, and some shampoos are hard on the hair, not to mention the dust, air pollution and chemicals in the air. Hair dyes contain harmful chemicals and not only penetrate the scalp but dry out the hair. The dyes can enter the blood stream and cause adverse reactions in the body. Lead is only one problem that arises from using hair dyes.

Dietary deficiency is something we can change to improve our hair health. It seems to be the last thing we think about when we have dull, receding hairlines, bald spots or undue loss of hair. The idea that nutritional deficiencies may be showing up in the conditions of the hair does not dawn on us.

Hair analysis is an effective tool to determine what is lacking in the body. It is respected as a way to determine toxic-metal poisoning in the body. Toxic metal measured by hair analysis are cadmium, lead, arsenic, mercury and aluminum to name a few.

Minerals are about 200 times more concentrated in the hair than they are in the blood, making them easier to measure accurately. Hair analysis reflects concentrations of toxic metals,revealing the buildup of these elements in the tissues. It will help determine mineral deficiencies in the body.

NATURAL THERAPY—Blood Purification, cleansing fast, using fresh vegetable juices (very rich in minerals). Stimulation therapy will help cleanse and bring nutrients to the scalp area. Olive oil and wheat germ oil are good for scalp stimulation. Hot and cold towels, alternating each for about twelve minutes will bring circulation to the head area. Colon cleanse will also help rid the body of toxins that contribute to hair loss. Make certain digestion is efficient enough for mineral assimilation.

Exercise helps to relax the entire body and mind. It increases circulation. The hair follicles need circulation for nourishment through the blood to stimulate hair growth.

FOODS TO HEAL—Herbal teas that help are rosemary, sage, nettle and oatstraw. Raw and steamed vegetables contain minerals, essential for hair health. Whole grains contain B vitamins for healthy hair. Grains, seeds, and nuts contain protein which is essential for healthy hair. It contains 95 to 98 percent protein. A variety of whole grains (thermos cooking), fruits and vegetables will improve the general condition of the hair.

VITAMINS AND MINERALS—Vitamin A protects against dry scalp, which can cause baldness. It is good for liver function. An unhealthy liver can result in hair loss. B-complex vitamins are essential for healthy hair. Lack of B1 can cause gray hair and hair loss. This vitamin helps in digestion, assimilation and elimination of food. Lack of B2 causes dull hair and loss of hair. B6 and pantothenic acid are good for gray hair; deficiency causes excessively oily skin and hair. B12 acts as a nutritional stimulant to prevent gray hair, loss of hair and dry scaly skin. Biotin and Choline and inositol work together to protect hair follicles. Vitamin C with bioflavonoids protect the immune system and works with B12 in the breakdown and utilization of protein. PABA and pantothenic acid help increase hair growth and natural color. Vitamin E improves circulation and helps to balance hormones which can cause hair loss.

All minerals are essential for healthy hair. Silicon and sulphur are essential for new hair growth. Calcium normalizes mineral metabolism. Chlorine, copper, fluorine, work with silicon for healthy hair. Iodine, Iron, Magnesium, Manganese, Potassium and zinc (deficiency can cause hair loss).

HERBAL COMBINATIONS—Blood Purifier, Bone, Female Problems formulas (balances hormones). Gland, Hair-Skin-Nail, Nerve, Stress.

SINGLE HERBS—Key herbs: Alfalfa (rich in minerals), Black Cohosh (balances hormones), Dulse (rich in minerals), Horsetail (rich in silicon), Jojoba (use oil it will clean and nourish the scalp), Kelp (rich in minerals), Licorice (helps adrenals), Oatstraw (rich in silicon), Parsley, Rosemary, Yarrow. Other important herbs: Comfrey, Pau D'Arco, Red Clover, Red Raspberry, Sarsaparilla, Slippery Elm, Watercress, Wormwood.

SUPPLEMENTS—Essential Fatty Acids (lack of can cause hair to fall out), Salmon Oil, Evening primrose Oil, Lecithin. Blue-green algae. Rice Bran Syrup, Chelated Cell Salts.

AVOID—Refined sugars and white flour products, rancid oils, ham, bacon, hot dogs, corned beef, lunch meats, alcohol, processed foods, fried foods and salt. These foods create stress on the body and deplete nutrients rapidly.

HALITOSIS
(bad breath)

Bad breath can be caused from diseases teeth or gums, chronically infected tonsils, sinuses or nasal infections, or even lung abscess, or bronchial disease.

The main cause of bad breath is constipation. The residue from food that is not digested properly can ferment and rot in the intestines and produce an odor. Regular bowel function is essential to avoid accumulation of waste and toxin products which can reabsorb into the bloodstream and disrupt the chemistry of the gastrointestinal tract. In the mornings, when the valves of the stomach are open, is when the smell is most prevalent. Many strange and strong odors can emanate from the gastrointestinal tract. Food that is not digested properly can create residues in the upper tract which cause bad odors.

Lack of hydrochloric acid in the stomach and lack of the normal mucus that coats the lining of the stomach can cause odors, especially in the elderly.

NATURAL THERAPY—Blood Purification and Bowel Cleansing Therapy are needed. Cleansing the intestinal tract for better absorption and elimination will improve bad breath. If the lungs are the problem, then deep breathing exercises will help clean the bottom of the lungs which are not always thoroughly cleansed. Chewing whole cloves and parsley will help bad breath.

FOOD TO HEAL—A cleansing diet, using all raw foods, especially raw fruit and vegetable juices.

VITAMINS AND MINERALS—Vitamins A, B-complex and C with bioflavonoids, and vitamin E will heal and protect from toxins accumulating in the body. A multi-mineral supplement with extra potassium, selenium and zinc.

HERBAL COMBINATIONS—Blood Purifier, Digestion, Liver, Lower Bowels.

SINGLE HERBS—Key herbs: Alfalfa, Aloe Vera (clean the digestive tract), Cascara Sagrada (cleans and strengthens the bowels), Cloves (sweetens the breath and helps in digestion), Kelp (rich in minerals), Golden Seal (cleans the digestive tract for better assimilation), Parsley (destroys odors), Peppermint (sweetens the breath and helps in digestion). Other vital herbs: Chaparral, Echinacea, Irish Moss, Myrrh, Watercress.

SUPPLEMENTS—Liquid Chlorophyll, Acidophilus, Green Drinks, Fresh Lemon Juice in pure water. Blue-green algae.

AVOID—Constipation, which will not only cause bad breath but create other diseases. Avoid all unnatural food: sugar (not a food), salt, meat, especially salted and preserved with additives. White flour products.

HAY FEVER

Millions of Americans suffer untold allergic reactions each spring and summer. It manifests itself in watery eyes, itching nose and eyes, runny nose, blurred vision, headaches, sinus aches and pains and a head that feels as big as a balloon. Red swollen eyes and difficulty in breathing are both common in hay fever. Tickling in the nose and throat are very irritating. Hay fever is like a very severe cold without any relief. It usually continues day after day, growing worse year after year, unless natural methods are used to help nature eliminate it through the natural way.

Hay fever is an inflammation of the nasal mucosa. Healthy mucus membranes protect all the organ linings from invasion by bacteria: when the mucus membranes are not healthy, the membranes are vulnerable to irritation by germs or any air borne irritant, and this irritation results in an increase of mucus flow which is out of control.

Hay fever and all other allergic reaction as well as acute diseases are acute catarrhal symptoms trying to clean and purify the body of toxins. It is an elimination of toxins by way of the mucus membranes.

Long before hay fever develops there is catarrh of the stomach, due to an abuse of overloading the stomach with overeating, wrong combinations and wrong kinds of food. It could also stem from too much rich food or holding within anger, hate, resentments or negative thoughts. We build up protein acids, starch acids, which create other acids from over-consumption of fried and rancid oils. These all cause irritations and inflammations of the stomach lining which lead to a chronic gastric fermentation. The gas from this fermentation is passed directly by way of the stomach and is also built up in the lungs. Conditions such as hay fever are primarily caused by the irritations from gas elimination (toxic) that is being generated in the stomach.

When the body is overloaded with too many toxins and trying to eliminate them from the natural eliminative organs (kidneys, colon or skin), the stress is then put on the lungs and nasal membranes. In trying to eliminate chronic catarrh hay fever develops. It may take years of the accumulation of toxins before hay fever develops or it can start with a baby born with toxins inherited from the parents.

NATURAL THERAPY—Blood Purification and Tonification Therapy are needed to clean and strengthen the body. Cleaning the blood and lower bowels will speed up the elimination of hay fever. Skin brushing will help eliminate gas and toxins from the skin. Foot Reflexology and Chiropractic treatments will speed circulation and healing.

FOODS TO HEAL—Green drink will help purify the blood. Raw diet and proper food combining will help in assimilation and elimination of food. Raw vegetable salads with sprouts. Sprouted grains. Wheat grass juice. Barley green drinks. Fresh fruit are cleansers of the body. Especially use short fasts using citrus juices. They are very cleansing.

VITAMINS AND MINERALS—Vitamin A protects and heals the mucus membranes. B-vitamins are depleted quickly in acute diseases. Pantothenic acid (essential in the production of cortisone).

Vitamin C with bioflavonoids (has a natural antihistamine effect). Vitamin E (helps suppress the release of histamines and prevents fluid accumulation outside the blood vessels).

Multi-mineral supplement—all minerals are essential for healing the body. Selenium, silicon and zinc are all necessary for healing.

HERBAL COMBINATIONS—Allergy, Blood Purifiers, Bone, Digestion, Lungs, Lower Bowels.

SINGLE HERBS—Key herbs: Burdock (cleans blood), Cayenne (improves circulation), Chaparral (cleans and eliminates toxins), Chickweed (soothing and healing for the respiratory system), Comfrey (cleans up dead tissues and restores new), Echinacea (builds up the immune system), Fenugreek (dissolves hardened mucus and expel toxins), Golden Seal (natural antibiotic and healer), Licorice (induces the adrenal glands to produce its own natural cortisone, provides strength to a weakened system). Lobelia (cleans the stomach), Ma Hueng (natural antihistamine), Marshmallow (contains antiseptic properties and is healing and soothing), Myrrh, Pau D'Arco (cleans liver for better elimination of toxins), Red Raspberry, Scullcap, Slippery Elm (high in nutrients such as calcium, zinc and vitamin C, and is healing), Yellow Dock. Other important herbs: Alfalfa, Aloe Vera, Dandelion (protects the liver), Eyebright, Gentian (heals the digestive tract), Hops, Irish Moss, Wood Betony, Wormwood.

SUPPLEMENTS—Bee Pollen, Acidophilus (milk free), Blue green algae. Essential fatty acids: Salmon Oil, Evening Primrose Oil, fish lipids.

AVOID—Milk and milk products (creates extra mucus), Meat, contains hormones, additives and antibiotics that create irritations. Wheat may sometimes cause problems (may not be digesting), use millet, brown rice, buckwheat or corn meal. Avoid white sugar products; they deplete vitamins and minerals for strengthening the mucus membranes.

HEADACHES
(also migraines)

In 1932, in a Medical Journal and Record one doctor wrote, "Headaches are among the most frequent complaints of human life."

Today headaches are still one of the most common complaints doctors see. It is believed that headaches in our modern day the price we pay for fast-paced living. It isn't true; headaches are as old as recorded history and as common in primitive societies as today. In ancient Melanesian, European and Meso-American societies it was believed that puncturing (called trephining) the skull to free evil spirits would cure persistent headaches, epilepsy or insanity. Skulls with trephining punctures go back ages to the Neolithic and Bronze ages.

An estimated 80 million Americans will suffer from headache pain and about 10 million will be afflicted with migraine. Thirty million pounds of aspirin are consumed each year in the United States.

Headaches are a symptom, not a disease. They come from poor dietary habits, lifestyle, environment, tension in the neck, shoulders or back, sinus as well as from brain tumors (less common).

Autointoxication headaches are the most common, and in the opinion of many health oriented doctors, originate from the stomach. Wrong food combinations, overeating and junk food will cause fermentation in the intestines and stomach. This cause gases, which enter the blood and causes irritation on the nerves and brain and causes headaches. Pressure in the temples and forehead usually indicate that there are stomach problems. Throbbing pain often results from congestion in the liver, spleen or digestive tract. Migraine headaches are caused by excess starches and sugars in the diet.

If the stomach, colon and mucus membranes were healthy, then allergic reactions to food wouldn't cause headaches. Stress, tension, constipation, sinusitis, head injury, air pollution, poor circulation and poor respiration are all causes of headaches. Allergies to MSG, chocolate, caffeine, wheat (pesticides), sulfites, sugar, dairy products, alcohol and vinegar can also cause headaches. An emotional conflict or anxiety can cause real headaches. High blood pressure can cause headaches.

Children with headaches often have eye problems, but they could be allergies, or emotional.

NATURAL THERAPY—Blood Purifiers and Lower Bowel Cleansers. Chiropractic treatments and foot reflexology will help normal nerve stimulation. Bones may be out of place. Tension in the jaws, neck or head can he helped by manipulation. Changing the diet to a more natural one using fresh vegetables and fruits. Whole grains, cooked thermos style for retention of B-vitamins and enzymes.

Cool cloth on the neck and head will relieve some headaches, while rest and relaxation will help others.

FOODS TO HEAL—Herbal teas: chamomile, mint and ginger. Pure water. Detoxify the body with fresh vegetable juices for healing and fruit juices for cleansing. Wheat grass juice, green drinks.

Change to a wholesome diet using grains, beans, fresh salads, steamed vegetables, seeds nuts and sprouts. They are healing and nourishing to the body.

VITAMINS AND MINERALS—Vitamin A (heal the mucus membranes), B-complex (with extra niacin, B15 and pangamic acid) will relax muscles. A deficiency of vitamin B5 or pantothenic acid results in headaches, and also depression. C with bioflavonoids (constricts and cleans veins), E, (increases oxygen in the blood).

Multi-mineral with extra calcium and magnesium (balance), potassium, iron and iodine. Zinc can give headache relief. All minerals are vital for health.

HERBAL COMBINATIONS—Allergy, Blood Purifier, Digestion, Glands, Lower Bowels, Nerve, Pain and Stress formulas.

SINGLE HERBS—Key herbs: Burdock (blood purifier), Cascara Sagrada, Chamomile, Dandelion (liver cleanser), Feverfew (helps in pain, especially in migraines), Golden Seal (helps clean the digestive tract where headaches can originate), Hops (relaxes nerves, calms pain), Horsetail (rich in minerals), Psyllium (cleans the colon), Red Clover (excellent blood cleanser), Scullcap (helps in pain), White Willow (pain reliever), Wood Betony (relieves pain). Other important herbs: Alfalfa, Aloe Vera, Black Cohosh, Black Walnut, Buchu, Buckthorn, Capsicum, Chaparral, Echinacea, Garlic, Ginger, Ginseng, Hawthorn, Ho Shou-Wu, Licorice, St. Johnswort, Uva Ursi, Yarrow, Yellow Dock, Yucca.

SUPPLEMENTS—Lecithin, Rice Bran Syrup, Evening Primrose Oil. External: Chinese Essential Oils, Tea Tree Oil. Salmon Oil, Spirulina, Blue-Green Algae.

AVOID—Constipation, wrong food combining. MSG, found in Chinese cooking. Sodium nitrate found in hot dogs. Nitrates and nitrites are used to preserve or cure meats: bacon, ham, salami, corned beef, and lunch meats. Caffeine can precipitate a headache.

Tyramine is a food chemical that dilates blood vessels and can cause headaches. Foods containing tyramine: Aged cheeses, pickled herring, salted dried fish, sausages, beef and chicken, liver, sauerkraut, vanilla, chocolate, yeast, some soy sauce, beer, ale, red wines. Nicotine can trigger a headache and can produce a "rebound headache".

HEMORRHOIDS
(Varicose Veins)

Hemorrhoids and varicose veins are caused from chronic constipation and circulatory system weakness. Liver congestion has been implicated as another cause. It is seen in pregnancy, junk food diet (clogs the circulatory system), lack of exercise, sitting while working, heavy lifting, and obesity. It is seen in low fiber diets.

Varicose veins occur most often in the legs. Weakness in the veins allows blood to accumulate and stretch the capillaries and veins and cause discoloring and tenderness and sometimes pain.

There are external hemorrhoids and internal hemorrhoids. External are easily identifiable and are usually more painful. Internal hemorrhoids may be present for years and not cause trouble. They can also appear externally if they become swollen and protrude the anal ring. Bleeding may be the first sign of internal hemorrhoids. Constant bleeding over a period of time can cause anemia.

If left untreated varicose veins can lead to phlebitis, leg ulcers, permanently swollen legs, pulmonary emboli (or clots in the lungs), and even surface leg hemorrhaging.

NATURAL THERAPY—Blood Purification, Circulatory Strengthening and Lower Bowel Cleansers will help in hemorrhoids and varicose veins. Liver cleansing to promote better filtering of toxins. A high fiber diet, using whole grains, fresh salads and vegetables (contain minerals for strengthening the veins). Use sprouted seeds and grains, and fresh fruits. Chewing food well and correct food combining will help assimilate and eliminate food properly. Use short fasts, using green drinks, wheatgrass juice and pure water.Carrot and celery juices are beneficial.

Exercise will strengthen the veins and increase circulation. Just walking if nothing else. It will help prevent deposits of clotting blood within the veins. Jogging, cycling, hiking will help prevent the tendency toward varicose veins.

Raw red potato or clove of garlic used as a suppository for hemorrhoids. Use several times a week. Sitz baths when continued for several days will help strengthen the veins. The sitz bath involves using two basins, one with hot water, and one cold. Use the hot basin first and cold last. The warm water relaxes the spasms of the muscles and the cold one tightens the tissues.

FOODS TO HEAL—Figs, raisins and prunes, soaked in pure water before using them. Citrus fruit, using the inner skin, will strengthen and heal the veins. Okra, rich in silicon and selenium, helps opens clogged veins and strengthen capillaries. Oat bran is very beneficial for keeping the veins clean. Buckwheat contains rutin, a bioflavonoid which strengthens the veins and decreases the tendency of the capillaries to break easily.

VITAMINS AND MINERALS—Vitamin A strengthens the veins. B-complex vitamins with extra B6, B12, B15 and choline and inositol found in lecithin. Vitamin C with bioflavonoids strengthens the veins and capillaries. Vitamin E is a vital nutrient for varicose veins. Protects the cells and veins from damage. Apply vitamin E externally also. Multi-mineral supplement with extra silicon and selenium (they will open up clogged veins and strengthen them). Zinc, calcium and vitamin D are very important in healing veins.

HERBAL COMBINATIONS—Blood Purifier, Bone, Chelation (clean the veins), Colitis, Digestion, Liver and Gallbladder, Lower Bowels.

SINGLE HERBS—Key herbs: Aloe Vera, Black Walnut (rich in minerals), Butcher's Broom (strengthens the blood vessels and keep them clean), Capsicum, Cascara Sagrada (colon rebuilder), Comfrey, Golden Seal, Horsetail (contains silicon), Kelp (strengthens and cleans veins). Mullein Oil (relieves pain), Oatstraw, Pau D'Arco (cleans the liver and protects the system), White Oak Bark (strengthens veins), Witch Hazel. Other vital herbs: Alfalfa, Bayberry, Buckthorn, Chaparral, Lobelia, Parsley, Red Raspberry, Slippery Elm, Uva Ursi, Wood Betony.

SUPPLEMENTS—Bee Pollen, Blue-green Algae, Glucomannan, Lecithin, Liquid Chlorophyll, Oak Bark Poultice, Psyllium, Spirulina. Salmon Oil, Germanium, Co Q10. Liquid mineral and herb drinks. Comfrey and Golden Seal ointment. Calendula ointment helps in itching and pain; Mullein oil also helps in pain. Wheatgrass poultices will stimulate healing of tissues. Clay packs will stimulate healing.

AVOID—Margarine (clogs veins), and all unnatural fats. Meat, especially beef. High sugar and white flour food. Candy, cookies, ice cream, pastries will clog up the veins.

HEPATITIS
(Liver Problems, Jaundice)

The medical term for hepatitis is "inflammation of the liver". Hepatitis A is a viral infection and is transmitted by food handling with unwashed hands by restaurant employees. It is also transmitted by saliva, semen, urine or by fecal contamination of water or food. Hepatitis B or serum hepatitis is mainly transmitted in hospitals by needles for drugs, transfusions and dialysis.

Robert S. Mendelsohn, M.D., states, "The incidence of hepatitis among the female technicians who perform renal dialysis is so high that some hospitals have removed the machines. But please note: where they are still in use, it isn't the male doctor who ordered the treatments who gets hepatitis; it is the female technician who handles the blood and operates the machines!" (Page 29, in MALE Practice, by Dr. Mendelsohn.)

The liver is the largest solid organ of the body and weighs about four pounds. The liver is also the detoxifier of the body. Everything we eat, drink, breathe and absorb through the skin is purified by the liver. Thousands of chemical reactions take place in the liver every second of our lives. Eighty percent of the liver can be destroyed and it will still keep us alive.

Toxic overload is the basic cause of liver problems. Our bodies can tolerate a certain amount of contamination. When the liver is overloaded, the toxins will circulate in the blood and can enter in the brain, nervous system or other organs and interfere with the normal functioning. Constipation is the main cause for the liver to be overloaded. When the liver tries to expel the poisons forced on it, it overloads the kidneys, for it is through the kidneys that the impurities are ultimately expelled.

Some of the signs of liver malfunction are: Yellowed complexion, Digestive disturbances, sluggish feeling in the mornings, Headaches (direct cause is constipation), Insomnia (sluggish liver effects the brain and nervous system),

Some of the functions of the liver are:

1. Controlling the production and elimination of cholesterol.

2. Maintaining hormone balance.

3. Regulating blood clotting.

4. Helping the body resist infection by producing immune factors and removing bacteria from the bloodstream.

5. Maintaining and monitoring the proper level of many chemicals and drugs in the blood.

6. Cleansing the blood and discharging waste products into the bile.

7. Neutralizing and destroying poisonous substances.

8. Regulating fat distribution.

9. Metabolizing alcohol.

10. Aiding the digestive process by producing bile.

11. Producing quick energy when it is needed.

12. Storing iron and other vitamins, minerals and sugars to prevent shortages when it is needed.

13. Manufacturing new body proteins.

14. It has the ability to regenerate its own damaged tissue.

NATURAL THERAPY—Blood Purification, Liver Purifiers and Lower Bowel therapy. The liver handles whatever we eat,so we need to protect it by giving it living food. Rest the liver with pure water and juice fasting. Use fresh lemon juice in warm water for a few days, fasting to restore liver function. Overeating is very hard on the liver. Lack of exercise can indirectly damage the liver by failing to stimulate the lungs to detoxify, causing an overburdened liver.

FOODS TO HEAL—Lemon juice, celery juice with a little carrot juice, rich in vitamin A for healing. Beet juice is healing. Eat lots of green vegetables and sprouts. Steamed vegetables, potassium broths (potato peelings, onions, carrot tops, celery), unsweetened yogurt. Raw seeds and nuts (make milk). Swiss chard, beet greens and celery. Green beans, spinach and onions. Strawberries, grapes and cherries are a tonic. Cold-pressed olive oil is cleansing and digestible for the liver. Grapefruit, oranges and avocados have a good influence on the liver.

Eat mostly raw foods. Eating overcooked foods places a strain on the liver as they do not supply live enzymes and amino acids vital for proper digestion.

VITAMINS AND MINERALS—Natural emulsion vitamin A (beta carotene) has to convert to vitamin A in liver which puts a strain. B-complex vitamins are essential for a healthy liver. B2 and B6 are essential for the breakdown and utilization of carbohydrates, fats and protein. Pantothenic acid is useful to fight stress along with folic acid. Use a liquid or maybe injections are necessary. Vitamin C with bioflavonoids (deficiency can cause severe liver degeneration); it protects the liver from damage. Vitamin E speeds healing and prevents scarring which is common in advanced stages of cirrhosis. Multi-mineral with extra calcium and magnesium (use herbal calcium), which are essential for blood clotting.

HERBAL COMBINATIONS—Kidney, liver and Gallbladder formulas, Digestion, Lower Bowels.

SINGLE HERBS—Key Herbs: Burdock (restores function of liver and gallbladder), Cascara Sagrada (heals liver), Dandelion (clears obstruction of the liver and detoxifies), Gentian (strong bitter, helps digestion and liver function), Golden Seal (helps regulate liver function), Licorice (combines well with bitters, to balance formulas), Milk Thistle (heals damaged liver), Pau D'Arco (protects the liver from further damage, strengthens the whole body), Parsley and Watercress (helps keep liver in balance), Saffron (digest fats to aid the liver and gallbladder), Wild Yam (removes toxic buildup of bile), Wormwood (stimulates the liver, eliminates worms), Yellow Dock (protects the liver, rich in iron for a healthy liver).

SUPPLEMENTS—Blue-green Algae, Chlorophyll, Germanium, Co Q10, Bentonite, Evening Primrose Oil, Salmon Oil, Glucomannan. Lecithin.

AVOID—Fried foods (very hard to digest). Drugs are very hard on the liver, especially sleeping pills, which will also destroy the nervous system. Avoid all refined foods, sugars and artificial sweeteners and caffeine drinks. Avoiding eating too much, which overburdens the liver. Artificial colorings, preservatives, flavorings and other chemicals overwork the liver. Devitalized food clogs the liver, causes impure blood and irritates the stomach and intestines.

HIATAL HERNIA

Hiatal Hernia is a very common disease which is estimated to affect fifty percent of the people over the age of forty. It is a bulging of the stomach above the diaphragm. This creates an opening in the diaphragm muscles which pushes part of the stomach up. Leakage of acid in the lower esophagus is the reason for the discomfort and burning feeling. It can be caused from a low fiber diet, constipation (straining for eliminations), lack of exercise (loss of muscle tone in stomach), eating wrong combinations of food (causes fermentation and gas that protrudes stomach upwards). Anger and hate have a profound negative effect on the stomach.

Symptoms are: Regurgitation of food—already digested food will come back up the esophagus and cause pain and a burning feeling. Nausea and lack of appetite, for fear of belching or regurgitating up food. Intestinal gas, constipation (can cause problems in the stomach), and vomiting (which can cause excess acid and spasms).

Many people are sleeping with pillows under their head to alleviate the condition. Many sleep in a recliner to get relief. Some people have surgery but this does not help the cause of hiatal hernia. The cause needs to be treated naturally for permanent relief.

If hiatal hernia isn't corrected it can causes serious problems to arise because of improper digestion and assimilation. Without nutritional support in the body from lack of assimilation, many things happen to the bones, glands, liver, pancreas and the entire intestinal tract. Ulcers are common with hiatal hernia. Many people have migraine headaches who have this problem. It affects the liver and creates problems with cholesterol that cannot be eliminated properly. Many problems arise with hiatal hernia that could be corrected.

Theodore A. Baroody, Jr.,D.C., gives us an exercise we can do to help ourselves. He says, "If there is shortness of breath, or the feeling that food is hung up and isn't going down properly, simply drink two 8 ounce glasses of water and bounce on the heels 12 times. First, this puts weight in the stomach, and the bouncing will jar it into place." His book Hiatal Hernia Syndrome: Insidious Link To Major Illness, gives us valuable information on self-healing.

NATURAL THERAPY—A Chiropractor can manipulate the hiatal hernia back where it belongs. Blood Purifiers, and Lower Bowel Cleansers will help purify and clean the system. A proper diet is essential, using proper food combining (to avoid fermentation and formation of gas and toxins). Keep meals small and simple. Exercise will help this ailment. *Hiatal Hernia Syndrome* by Theodore A. Baroody, Jr. M.A., D.C., describes proper diet and exercises to help yourself. Avoid using liquids with meals; it dilutes hydrochloric acid which is essential in digestion of food. A loving, positive attitude is a must for a healthy stomach.

FOODS TO HEAL—Raw nuts (almonds), seeds (sesame, sunflower, pumpkin), and figs and raisins (soak first), you can also soak nuts to make milk drinks. Apples and fresh apple juice, grapes, plums, peaches, bananas, pineapple. Unsweetened juices: cranberry, cherry and raspberry. Vegetables: asparagus, avocados, beets, broccoli, cabbage, cauliflower, carrots, celery, cucumbers, peas, radishes, squash, string beans, tomatoes. Potatoes, raw and baked. Fresh green salads, using leaf lettuce and lots of fresh vegetables. Brown rice, millet and buckwheat are healing and easy to digest.

VITAMINS AND MINERALS—Vitamin A is very healing; B-complex vitamins are essential for a healthy stomach and digestion. Vitamin C with bioflavonoids are healing and cleansing. Multi-minerals with extra calcium and magnesium, potassium, sodium (in herbs), selenium, silicon and zinc are healing.

HERBAL COMBINATIONS—Blood Purifiers, Bone (rich in minerals), Colitis formulas, Digestion, Glands, Immune formulas, Lower Bowels, Nerve and Ulcer formulas.

SINGLE HERBS—Key herbs: Alfalfa, Aloe Vera (healing), Capsicum, (healing and creates circulation), Comfrey and Pepsin, Gentian (healing and strengthening for digestive system), Ginger, Golden Seal (excellent for healing), Hops, Horsetail, Marshmallow, Papaya, Scullcap, Slippery Elm (healing and provides needed protein). Other helpful herbs: Black Walnut, Burdock, Echinacea, Garlic, Hawthorn, Yellow Dock, Yucca.

SUPPLEMENTS—Blue-green Algae, Liquid Chlorophyll, Aloe Vera Juice (Use a combination of Comfrey, Golden Seal, Slipper Elm and Aloe Vera and mix with apple juice and drink slowly for healing), CoQ10, Germanium, Evening Primrose Oil, Salmon Oil, Glucomannan, Lecithin.

AVOID—Alcohol, soft drinks, all sugar products (candy, cookies, cake, pie, ice cream), all caffeine drinks, refined white flour products: spaghetti, macaroni, noodles and white rice.

HERPES
(Simplex and Genital Herpes)

Type I is called simplex and is recognized as cold sores and skin eruptions. It is most common on the mouth, on the lips, in the eyes. Type II is genital herpes and is sexually transmitted and is very contagious. Herpes II virus in women increases the chance of premature delivery or miscarriage. The baby could also be infected. It can cause brain, blindness or neurological damage. Herpes is a virus that is originally caused by skin-to-skin contact. Herpes can lay dormant and than recur, when the immune system is lowered through stress, diet, autointoxication, a feverish illness, overexposure to sunlight, some foods and drugs. The initial infection can go away but not the virus. Herpes hangs on, lodging itself in a dormant state in the skin or nervous system.

It usually starts with a brief period of itching or tingling, when you realize what you have. A blister will than appear with small blisters and persist for several days before they begin to dry, forming a yellowish crust. Healing takes about a week to 10 days, and maybe even three weeks. With natural treatment it can be healed in a shorter period.

NATURAL THERAPY—Blood Purification and Nervine Therapy, also Lower Bowel Cleansing. A cleansing diet is essential to restore the body to its normal balance. Use more alkaline foods to start with. Too much acid food will trigger herpes. Herpes is a cleansing of the body, nature's method of cleansing impurities from the system for a healthier lifestyle. Don't suppress herpes; use natures remedies to eliminate the herpes virus. Short fasts, using fresh vegetable juices will help.

Daily exercise in the fresh air will build the immune system and increases resistance to disease. Learning to deal with stress and have a calm, loving attitude without anger, frustration and hate will also help.

FOODS TO HEAL—Whole grains (thermos cooking), beans and steamed vegetables. Fresh fruit, vegetables and sprouts. Fresh fish, canned fish, chicken, goat's milk. Food combining is very important. Drink pure water, vegetable and fruit juices, and herbal teas. Limit protein, especially red meat; it is very hard to digest. Chew food well; this is easier on the digestive system for better healing and building.

VITAMINS AND MINERALS—Vitamin A is essential for healing the mucus membranes. Vitamin C with bioflavonoids, is also healing . B-complex vitamins (yeast free). Vitamin E is healing. Multi-minerals with extra calcium and magnesium (herbal calcium), selenium and zinc are healing and protects the immune system.

HERBAL COMBINATIONS—Blood Purifiers, Bone, Candida, Colitis, Digestion, Immune, Infection formulas and Lower Bowels and Stress formulas.

SINGLE HERBS—Aloe Vera (fresh and powdered), Black Walnut (external and internal), Comfrey, Garlic, Golden Seal (heals), Myrrh, Oregon Grape, Pau D'Arco (cleans blood), Red Clover, Rose Hips, Slippery Elm (heals mucus membranes).

SUPPLEMENTS—Acidophilus, Blue-green algae, Evening Primrose Oil, Salmon Oil, Lecithin, Spirulina, Tea Tree Oil (external).
L-Lysine.

AVOID—Chocolate, corn, peanuts, walnuts. All nuts can trigger herpes. Avoid alcohol, processed foods, all white sugar and white flour products (no food value anyway), cola and caffeine drinks, coffee.

HIGH BLOOD PRESSURE
(Hypertension)

Hypertension is a disease that involves the heart and the arteries that carry fresh blood to every part of the body. It's a major killer that causes stroke, heart disease, kidney disease and other problems. Hypertension occurs when cholesterol plaques and deposits in the walls of the arterioles harden and constrict these blood vessels, compressing the blood into a smaller volume and thereby raising its pressure. Hypertension is also manifested neurologically when emotional stress triggers the response to "fight or flight" response. This causes the muscles to squeeze these tiny blood vessels; they compress the blood into a smaller volume, which then raises the pressure.

It's a degenerative disease caused by incorrect living habits, eating and attitude towards living. We need to understand ourselves and why we act the way we do. We need to deal with stress and tensions in our lives. Only we can do it for ourselves. The body needs to be fortified nutritionally first, before we can even think properly. Strengthening the nervous system should be the first priority when dealing with stress.

This disease can be reversed only if we take control of our lives and change our eating and living habits. Exercise more, watch our weight, avoid alcohol, tobacco and drugs of all kinds.

The body can heal itself. It takes dedication and commitment in order to succeed.

Chiropractic treatment is another way to determine if there is pinched nerves or subluxation that interfere with circulation and proper nerve function.

NATURAL THERAPY—Blood Purification, Lower Bowel Therapy and Nervine therapy will help in blood pressure. Short fasts will help reduce high blood pressure, using celery, parsley and cucumber juices. Parsley is a natural diuretic. Doctors usually put you on diuretics immediately. Exercise helps to reduce the body's reaction to nervous stress. A combination of diet changes and exercise will show an improvement quickly. Exercise should start gradually and work up to more.

FOODS TO HEAL—High fiber foods (whole grains, oat bran, beans, peas, vegetables and fruits), Potassium-rich food are fruits, vegetables and unsalted nuts. Lentils, oatmeal, brown rice and whole grain pasta. Green leafy vegetables, potatoes skins, bananas, oranges, sunflower seeds, nuts, raw garlic are all high in potassium.

VITAMINS AND MINERALS—Multi-vitamin with extra A and C with bioflavonoids, K, E (start slowly). Multi-minerals, with extra calcium (herbal formulas); magnesium, manganese, silicon, selenium, sodium (natural) and zinc. Potassium and sodium will help reduce high blood pressure and avoid cardiovascular disease.

HERBAL COMBINATIONS—Heart and Blood Pressure formulas, Glands, Nerves, Bone Combination, Chelation, Digestion, Lower Bowel.

SINGLE HERBS—Key herbs: Garlic (lowers blood pressure), Hawthorn (strengthens the veins), Hops (relaxes veins and nerves), Passion Flower (nerve relaxer), Parsley (natural diuretic), Pau D'Arco (blood cleanser), Scullcap (calms the nerves), Valerian (relaxer). Other vital herbs: Alfalfa, Aloe Vera, Black Cohosh, Capsicum (cleans the veins), Dandelion (cleans the liver), Echinacea (helps eliminate toxins from the veins), Ginger, Ginseng (strengthens the body), Gotu Kola (feeds the brain), Lady's Slipper, Mistletoe, Yarrow, Yellow Dock.

SUPPLEMENT—Liquid Chlorophyll, Lecithin, Salmon Oil, Evening Primrose Oil, Germanium, Co Q10, Glucomannan. Blue-green algae (enhances oxygen utilization). L-Carnitine helps to lower cholesterol, cleans veins and heart.

AVOID—Red meats; all meat at first, puts too much stress on the veins as well as hard to digest. Avoid salt, sugar, white flour products. Alcohol, caffeine drinks, cookies, candy, pastries.

Avoid a high fat diet, fats circulating in the blood, they begin to adhere to each other and grow. This creates plaque and sticky masses of material. These deposit on the vessel walls, become brittle and inhibit blood circulation. This hard material can break off and float around and cause a stroke or heart attack, by blocking the flow of blood and oxygen.

HYPERACTIVITY

Hyperactivity is commonly seen in children, but I have seen adults that suffer with this problem. It causes major difficulties and frustration in many homes in America. I feel that hypoglycemia in adults is an extension of hyperactivity in children. Many adults cannot cope with life's problems and take tranquilizers and drugs that only complicate the problems and cause a frustrating family life. It is felt that it is so common and puts such a stress on families that it can lead to divorce, marital difficulties and even child abuse. The term Hyperactivity is being replaced by "attention deficit disorder".

Seventy-five percent of criminals were hyperactive children; more than half have abnormal glucose tolerance tests. Diet and criminal behavior, hyperactivity and hypoglycemia are connected. A high percentage of hyperactive children grow up to be troubled teenagers: suicide, drugs, dropouts, crimes, depression, etc. A bad diet is seen in all three. It could be allergies, which is created from bad eating habits. It stems from nutritional deficiencies. Too much sugar leaches nutrients from the body. In fact nutrition is the number one problem of hyperactive children, as well as adults.

Symptoms of hyperactivity are: child squirms and fidgets, cannot sit still very long; attention span is short; runs instead of walks. They are into everything, and they talk constantly with a loud voice. They are impulsive, act before thinking and they forget easily. Have trouble following instructions and are often moody, irritated and indifferent when disciplined. They throw temper tantrums and are determined to get their way. These are a few of the symptoms.

Ritalin is widely prescribed for hyperactive children. This drug is not the answer. This drug is being used on more than a million children for the comfort and convenience of parents and teachers. Dr. Mendelsohn said, "You can expect your doctor to cast a covetous eye on your kids. Educators who don't like unruly pupils have, with the willing help of doctors and psychologists, broadened the definition of hyperactivity to include a substantial percentage of those in the country who are under age twenty-one. As a consequence, for the comfort and convenience of teachers and parents, millions of normally lively kids have been drugged with Ritalin and turned into virtual zombies by its effects."

NATURAL THERAPY—Lower Bowel cleansing and Blood Purifiers. The bowels, when not kept clean and eliminating every day will accumulate toxins in the blood and the brain and nervous system are very sensitive to these poisons. Keep food colorings, preservatives, sweets from those prone to hyperactivity. A hair analysis will determine whether there is heavy metal poisoning in the body. Children are very prone to cadmium and lead contamination.

FOODS TO HEAL—Food high in B-complex vitamins: Whole grains (thermos cooking to retain vitamins and enzymes), Buckwheat, millet, wheat, cornmeal, barley, and brown rice. Sunflower seeds, almonds, wild rice, brewer's yeast, molasses, wheat and oat bran, soybeans, egg yolk, sprouts, green leafy vegetables.

VITAMINS AND MINERALS—Vitamin A (protects against allergies), B-complex vitamins with extra B5, B6, B12 and niacin, Vitamin C with bioflavonoids. Multi-minerals with extra calcium, magnesium, selenium and zinc.

HERBAL COMBINATIONS—Allergies, Bone, Glands, Immune, Lower Bowel, Nervine, Stress.

SINGLE HERBS—Key herbs: Black Walnut (kills parasites), Burdock (cleans blood), Catnip (relaxing), Dandelion (cleans liver), Gotu Kola (brain food), Hops, Lady's Slipper (relaxes), Lobelia, Red Clover, Scullcap (builds nerves), Wood Betony. Other important herbs: Alfalfa, Chaparral, Chickweed, Echinacea, Golden Seal, Yellow Dock, Yucca.

SUPPLEMENTS—Bee Pollen, Blue-green algae, Rice bran syrup, Essential fatty acids: Salmon Oil, Evening Primrose Oil, Flaxseed Oil (not rancid), or whole flaxseed soaked in water.

AVOID—All sugar products, white flour products, soft drinks, salt, meat, hot dogs, lunch meats, preservatives and food colorings. Watch all food labeling and use only pure foods.

HYPERTHYROID AND HYPOTHYROID

Hyperthyroidism is when the thyroid gland produces too much thyroxine hormone, which results in an overactive metabolism. Hypothyroid is when the thyroid gland produces too little hormone. Symptoms of hyperthyroidism are: irritability, weakness, intolerance, rapid heartbeat, fatigue, insomnia, sweating, etc.

Symptoms of hypothyroid are (and the symptoms are frequently missed because they can be associated with other diseases): muscle cramps, low back pain, anemia, easy bruising, fatigue, P.M.S., hair loss, muscle weakness, recurrent infections, depression, a cold feeling. Shortage of vitamins C and E can bring on hyperthyroidism. In fact it is possible to correct unbalanced thyroid hormone production whether it be too much or too little by correcting vitamin and mineral deficiencies. We are talking about both thyroid imbalances. All glands are involved when one gland is in trouble. Essential fatty acids deficiency causes an unbalanced thyroid. Evening Primrose Oil has helped many people with this disease. Any essential fatty acid will improve symptoms.

The following is a self-test developed by Dr. Broda O. Barnes, M.D.: Take a thermometer and shake it down and put it on your bedstand. Immediately upon awakening in the morning, place the thermometer snugly in the armpit for ten minutes by the clock. A reading below the normal range of 97.8 to 98.2 strongly suggests low thyroid function. If the reading is above the normal range, one must be suspicious of some infection or an overactive thyroid gland.

NATURAL THERAPY—Blood Purifiers, Lymphatics Cleansing, Lower Bowel Cleansers. Raw foods are necessary for the glandular system. Cooked food kills the enzymes and causes the endocrine glands to become overworked and leads to body autoxidation and causes diseases such as hypothyroidism and hyperthyroidism.

Cooked foods over-stimulate the gland and cause the body to retain excess weight. The enzymes from live food help the body to maintain proper metabolism.

The problem arises when the glands do not receive the nutrients necessary to satisfy the body's needs. When this happens the glands overstimulate the digestive organs and demand more food (because the body is not satisfied). This produces an oversecretion of hormones and an unhealthy appetite, which finally results in exhaustion of the hormone-producing glands.

FOODS TO HEAL—Live foods, sprouts, salads, raw fruit and vegetables. Thermos cooked grains and rice, to retain the enzymes which heal and feed the glands. Seeds, nuts, such as sesame seeds, pumpkin, sunflower, and nuts such as almonds, pecans, cashews (raw and unsalted). Seaweeds are very nourishing to the glands. Raw vegetable juices (carrot, celery, parsley, comfrey), and green drinks containing chlorophyll for healthy blood.

VITAMINS AND MINERALS—Vitamin A assists in maintaining normal glandular function. B-complex vitamins are necessary to help control glandular health. They build the adrenals, thyroid and calm the nerves. Extra B3, B5, B6, B12, PABA. Vitamin C deficiency is seen in thyroid problems. Promotes normal adrenal function and glandular activity. Vitamins D and E work with vitamin A. E is essential for glandular health—protects the B vitamins from rapid oxidation. Vitamin F (essential fatty acids), a must for glandular health. It improves overall health. Multi-mineral, all minerals are involved in glandular health, calcium and magnesium, supports the glands, manganese, selenium, silicon and zinc protects the glands.

HERBAL COMBINATIONS—Blood Purifiers, Bone, Digestion, Glands, Immune, Nervine, Stress.

SINGLE HERBS—Adrenals: Licorice (stimulates the glands), Rose Hips (rich in Vitamin C and B-vitamins), Capsicum, Ginseng (strengthens the body). Pituitary: Alfalfa, Licorice, Ginseng, Gout Kola and Ho Shou-Wu. Thyroid: Black Walnut, Walnut, Kelp, White Oak Bark. Female glands: Black Cohosh, Dong Quai,

Damiana, Yellow Dock. Male Glands: Ginseng, Kelp, Damiana. Other vital herbs: Bayberry, Blue Cohosh, Burdock, Chaparral, Dandelion, Garlic, Ginger, Hawthorn, Hops, Kelp, Lobelia, Mistletoe, Parsley, Sarsaparilla (stimulates glandular function), Scullcap, Valerian, Wood Betony, Yellow Dock.

SUPPLEMENTS—Evening Primrose Oil, Linseed Oil, Bentonite Cleanse, Golden Seal, Echinacea.

AVOID—All junk food. They overstimulate the glands and cause exhaustion and weakness. Sugar and white flour products. Fried foods are hard to digest and cause free radicals to form and destroy the cells. Avoid all drugs: The Pill, antibiotics, sulfa drugs and tranquilizers. They will put a burden on the glands and cause dysfunction.

HYPOGLYCEMIA

Hypoglycemia means low blood sugar. Hypo means "low" and glycemia means "sugar". It is associated with "highs" and"lows". Moods swing drastically, from feeling happy and energetic to being anxious, irritable, tearful and depressed with mental confusion and manifestation of phobias.

Hypoglycemia is seen as the first step on the road to chronic degenerative disease because of its devastating effect on the body, especially in the stress-related adrenals. When one gland is weakened it has an effect on all the glands. It has a wear-and-tear effect on the body. It affects the nervous system, muscles and cells, as well as all the glands.

Dr. Robert Atkins, one of the foremost pioneers in the field of blood sugar disturbances says, "without improper nutrition, I don't believe diabetes could develop, even if both parents are diabetic. No one is doomed by heredity to develop diabetes, I also feel that we are not doomed to develop hypoglycemia or many of the diseases plagued by mankind, just because our parents have it."

The symptoms of hypoglycemia are very subtle to the person who has it. I have observed many people with hypoglycemia and their actions become so normal to them that they do not realize they are acting in a very negative and unusual way. Their way of perceiving and reacting to situations becomes distorted. One friend of mine went through a very traumatic period in her life. She knew that if she divorced her husband all her problems would be solved. Later when she was able to get her hypoglycemia under control, she realized that it wasn't her husband at all, it was she who was creating the problems.

Common symptoms: Anxiety, antisocial behavior, confusion, depression, emotional instability, exhaustion, headaches, impatience, inability to cope, intense hunger, phobias, sugar craving.

There are several causes of hypoglycemia which stem from a diet high in refined food and excessive sugar intake. Stress, glandular dysfunction and mineral deficiencies are also factors. The typical American diet is high in processed food, food chemically treated, overcooked, stripped of nutrients, sweetened and salted and altered in many ways. Fried foods are found in a typical diet and disrupt the glandular system.

Sugar is added to food products to increase consumption. Sugar is a very addictive substance; the low blood sugar state which you get from eating it makes you crave more. The food industry has discovered that increasing the sugar in a product also increases the amount a person will eat, which will increase sales. White sugar is not a food; it is a chemical which wears out the glandular system.

NATURAL THERAPY—Glandular therapy using herbs to strengthen and cleanse the glands. Frequent meals using wholesome food. Since fasting is hard on hypoglycemia, use cleansing drinks and lower bowel formulas to help clean the cells and colon, and liver. Parsley, wheatgrass, carrot and celery juices along with green vegetables build the blood.

Chiropractic or reflexology treatments are excellent to help control hypoglycemia along with diet, herbs, vitamins and minerals. Along with stress management and exercise.

FOODS TO HEAL—Sprouts will heal the glands: alfalfa, radish, mung beans, buckwheat, and fenugreek are excellent. Eat a variety of nourishing foods. Steamed and fresh vegetables, fresh fruit, a little to start with. Fish, chicken (organically grown), rice, baked potatoes. Thermos cooked grain and soups.

VITAMINS AND MINERALS—Vitamin A is healing for the glands. B-complex is a must (with extra B1, B3, B5, B6, B12, pantothenic acid), Vitamin C with bioflavonoids, and vitamin E. Multi-minerals (essential for glandular healing). Calcium, magnesium potassium, phosphorus, manganese, iodine, chromium and zinc.

HERBAL COMBINATIONS—Allergies, Bone, Digestion, Endurance, Glands, Hypoglycemia formulas, Immune, Nerves.

SINGLE HERBS—Alfalfa (nourishes the glands), Black Cohosh, Cayenne (aids in circulation of blood, which brings oxygen and other nutrients to cells in need of repair), Dandelion, Garlic, Ginger (stimulates blood and cleans capillaries), Gotu Kola (stimulates brain and relieves fatigue), Hawthorn (strengthens the heart when under stress), Juniper Berries, Kelp (cleans and nourishes the glands), Lady's Slipper, Licorice (feeds the adrenals and provides energy), Lobelia and Mullein are perfect glandular food, Parsley, Saffron (helps digest oils), Scullcap, Uva Ursi.

SUPPLEMENTS—Bee Pollen, Chlorophyll, Green Drinks, Royal Jelly, Lecithin, Spirulina, Wheatgrass juice. Essential fatty acids: Evening Primrose Oil, Salmon Oil or Flaxseed Oil.

AVOID—All sugar products, even fruit juices (too concentrated). Small amounts of fruit can be eaten (they are cleansing to the body). Avoid all unnatural food (fried, canned, or overcooked). Avoid alcohol, tobacco, high protein and fat diet, and stimulating food.

IMMUNE SYSTEM

Our immune system is in great danger from the widespread use of drugs. Tranquilizers, antibiotics and vaccinations are creating so-called "immune related diseases". Dr. Robert Mendelsohn said, "There is a growing suspicion that immunization against relatively harmless childhood disease may be responsible for the dramatic increase in autoimmune disease since mass inoculations were introduced."

The key to prevention and treatment of diseases is a healthy, well-functioning immune system. This wonderful apparatus we were born with is not the source of protection it once was. The body can be weakened to the point that it does not respond to the normal intake of nutrients. The immune system can accumulate damage, become defective and, consequently, cannot do its job. This problem plays a role in most degenerative diseases.

The immune system is genetically-programmed to shelter you from disease. It will protect you if you keep it in top shape. The immune system is equipped with glands, cells, organs, and proteins to fight off autoimmune diseases. With all of the diseases in the world ready to invade your body, your immune system must be prepared to battle these scourges.

IMMUNE RELATED DISEASES

AIDS—A devastating disease that alters the body's ability to protect itself. A complete breakdown of the immune system is the result. It is reaching epidemic proportions. Innocent women and babies are being infected. The AIDS virus, along with over forty more viruses, are found in the kidney of the Green African Monkey, of which vaccinations are made.

ANKYLOSING SPONDYLITIS—A disease Norman Cousins had and whipped. It is a progressive, inflammatory arthritis characterized by fusion of various joints, especially of the spine. He said that he was literally falling apart. His connective tissues were coming unglued.

BACTEREMIA—This is when bacteria invades the blood. It can come from any infection such as an abscess, or inflamed urinary tract, female organs, lung infections, intravenous drug use, urinary catheters, surgical procedures, or from any bacteria which get into the blood. When the blood is impure it creates infection anywhere.

CANCER—A breakdown in the body's immune system. Bad eating habits, impure blood and constipation can cause autointoxication where the toxins circulate in the bloodstream and invade the weakest part of the body.

CANDIDA ALBICANS—A yeast invader, which weakens the immune system. It is in epidemic proportions. This disease can produce mild symptoms or create pain, fatigue, and mental anguish. This is created by the medical profession who so freely prescribed antibiotics. Doctors are now realizing that antibiotics should not be given freely but now they are given to animals in their feed, assuring a constant supply of them in our food.

CHYLAMYDIAL DISEASES—A very common sexually transmitted disease that is increasing in epidemic proportions. It is serious because it can cause infertility in women, along with constant urinary tract and prostatic infection in men.

CRIB DEATH (Sudden Infant Death Syndrome)—Each year thousands of babies between four weeks and seven months of age die in their sleep. It is a heartbreaking disease for parents to find their precious baby lifeless. Crib death may result from a breakdown in the babies' immune systems. Babies are born with naturally low immunity, but acquire a certain amount from their mothers' antibodies in the placenta. SIDS is preponderately a disease which affects artificially fed infants. Bottle-fed babies suffer from deficiencies in oxygen. This causes bacteria to become pathogenic, parasitic and virulent. Virulent bacteria produces viruses which exhaust vitamin C and A, and minerals in the body.

EPSTEIN-BARR VIRUS (EBV)—This is a disease that is considered a cancer-triggering virus. This virus is found in the kidney of the African Green Monkey, which is used in vaccinations. This virus was once thought to be harmless but is now known to play a leading role in a deadly and horribly disfiguring cancer that strikes the noses and throats of some fifty thousand people a year. It has been associated with an immune cell cancer (Burkitt's lymphoma) that is usually found in children. This disease is devastating peoples' lives.

GASTRITIS—This is a superficial inflammation of the stomach lining. It is caused by drugs, stress (the stomach is the seat of our emotions), alcohol, and also caused by toxins recirculating in our blood stream because of autointoxication. Aspirin, cortisone, antibiotics and nonprescription drugs can wear away at our stomach lining. This can become chronic and cause serious problems such as ulcers or cancer if it is not taken care of.

LEGIONNAIRES' DISEASE—This is another disease caused by a breakdown in the immune system. It occurs more often in persons who are middle-aged to elderly, who have lymphoma or other disorders. It receives its name from the peculiar, highly publicized illness that struck 182 people (29 of whom died), at an American Legion convention in Philadelphia the summer of 1976. It is an acute bronchopneumonia produced by a gram-negative bacillus. It was found in the air conditioning in the building where the meeting was held. Again, the immune system plays a vital role in protecting one from this sickness.

LUPUS ERYTHEMATOSUS—Systemic. An autoimmune disease that usually strikes young women. One women I know who has Lupus was plagued with anorexia and bulimia for eight years, which has a devastating effect on the immune system. This is a connective tissue disease which causes inflammation. This is a disease where the body's own immune system attacks itself.

There are two kinds of Lupus. Discoid Lupus is much less serious, which affects the skin. Both kinds need nutrients and a healthy diet to keep it under control.

REYE'S SYNDROME—This is a childhood disease which targets children under 18. Parents have been warned not to give their children aspirin if they are suspected of having chicken pox or the flu. This combination seems to precipitate the syndrome. One group of children in Canada developed Reye's Syndrome after suffering from an influenza viral infection. This disease produces fever, vomiting and disturbance of consciousness progressing to coma and convulsions. It causes fatty infiltration of the liver and kidney's, with cerebral edema and many other destructive effects. A weakened immune system will promote susceptibility to this unfortunate problem.

TOXIC SHOCK SYNDROME—This disease affects menstruating women in their late teens or early twenties. It afflicts those who use highly absorbent synthetic fiber tampons, which are thought to trigger Staphyloccus Aures. This organism produces the toxins which cause Toxic Shock Syndrome. It is felt that one cause could be the absorbing effect depleting the body of magnesium, which protects the immune system. Many women have been stricken by this disease quite suddenly. In 1985 it was reported over the news that 114 women had died from this disease. These women usually experienced nausea, diarrhea, and dizziness, accompanied by a sudden high fever. This was often followed by a rash, peeling skin, and possibly shock, unconsciousness, paralysis and even death. A sharp drop in blood pressure is another symptom of this syndrome. Recovery is often a long and painful process.

NATURAL THERAPY—Blood Purifiers, Lower Bowel Cleaners, Nervine therapies to keep the immune system strong. The nervous system is connected to the immune system and when one is weakened the other one becomes weak. Change to a healthy diet, all nutrients affect the immune system. Exercise often. Do not let stressful situations control how you act. Fresh, clean air is vital for the lungs and immune system. Create happiness, love, and peace within yourself.

FOODS TO HEAL—Fish, vegetables such as broccoli, cabbage, cauliflower, brussels sprouts, parsley, chicken, apples, apricots, bananas, green beans, berries, cherries, corn, leaf lettuce (lots of salads), melons, okra, peaches, fresh peas, potatoes, prunes, plums, watercress, sprouts, brown rice, millet, buckwheat, pineapple, yellow cornmeal, rye, goat's milk.

VITAMINS AND MINERALS—The following three vitamins are important for many reasons. However, they are most famous for their antioxidant qualities which protects the immune system. Vitamin A increases resistance to infections and protects against pollution, cancer and viral infections. Vitamin E prevents the oxidized state that cancer cells thrive in. It deactivates the free radicals that promote cellular damage leading to malignancy. Vitamin C can activate white blood cells to battle foreign substances and increase the production of interferon, the body's antivirus protein. B-complex vitamins are vital, protects the nervous system, prevents fatigue, increases resistance to disease.

Multi-minerals with extra selenium and zinc manifests anti-carcinogenic (anti-cancer) and anti-mutagenic (prevents disorders leading to birth defects) properties. Selenium inhibits breast, skin, liver, and colon cancer. It is lost in food processing. Zinc is vital for the immune system. It produces histamine, which dilates the capillaries so that blood, carrying immune-fighting white blood cells, can hurry to the scene of an infection. Other important minerals are: Calcium (prevents heavy metals from accumulating in the body). Magnesium produces properdin, a blood protein that fights invading viruses and bacteria. Manganese, activates enzymes that work with vitamin C. Also use Iodine, iron, chromium.

HERBAL COMBINATIONS—Blood Purifiers, Bone, Candida, Digestion, Glands, Immune formulas, Lower Bowels, Nerves.

SINGLE HERBS—All herbs are good for the immune system. Key herbs: Burdock (blood cleanser), Ginkgo (helps in circulation), Ginseng (strengthens the whole body), Golden Seal (a great cleanser and healer), Capsicum (cleans the veins), Chaparral (great cell cleanser), Echinacea (lymphatic and blood cleanser), Garlic (antibiotic properties), Kelp, Lobelia, Mullein, Pau D'Arco (cleans blood and protects the liver), Red Clover, Suma, Watercress.

SUPPLEMENTS—Acidophilus, Bee Pollen, Blue-green algae, Essential fatty acids are vital to overall health. Evening Primrose Oil, Flaxseeds, Salmon Oil, Fish Oils, Spirulina.

AVOID—Alcohol, tobacco, drugs of all kinds. Tranquilizers (destroy the immune system). All sugar products, white flour products (no food value and depletes vital nutrients).

IMPOTENCE

Impotence is the inability to achieve or maintain an erection. In can develop because of mental and physical fatigue and stress. Being under constant pressure can lead to impotence. There are medications that can cause this problem. Anti-depressants, tranquilizers, anti-hypertensive drugs, and anti-ulcer drugs are some examples of medications which can cause impotence.

Tension will create the inability to perform by reducing blood flow to vessels of the male organ. Anxiety, fatigue, depression, unhappiness, marital problems, anger, hate and a poor self-image can all contribute to impotence.

I believe that nutritional deficiency and autointoxication are two very real causes of this problem. Proper circulation without cholesterol build-up in the veins is important. A positive mental outlook can be achieved when good health habits are implemented.

NATURAL THERAPY—Blood Purifying, Build up the Nerves, Lower Bowel Cleansing to eliminate toxic build-up in the body. Exercise to help with blood circulation and build a healthy heart. Try to achieve a good self-image through a proper attitude. No one else should be responsible for the way you feel. Create love, happiness and joy through nutrition and a healthy mental outlook.

FOODS TO HEAL—Fruit is important; they are cleansers of the body. Apples, oranges, lemons, grapefruit, bananas, papaya, grapes, cherries and all kinds of berries. Peaches, pears and apricots are good. Whole grains (contains essential minerals, such as zinc, selenium, manganese, copper, chromium), all necessary for a healthy sex life. Sprouts contain live enzymes (heat kills enzymes). I think seeds are important because they can create living food and therefore are good for the body. Beans, lentils, and peas are all good food.

VITAMINS AND MINERALS—Lack of Vitamin A will cause sterility and loss of vitality and vigor. It is essential for a healthy and strong body. B-complex vitamins (with extra B3, B4, B6, B12, folic acid and PABA), prevents nervous disorders, nutritional stimulant, utilizes energy in the brain and nervous system and protect against stress. Vitamin C with bioflavonoids, vital for all around health, prevents cholesterol from building up in the veins and protects against stress. The are vital for immune function and protect against viruses and germs. Vitamin E is called the "fertility vitamin." It is essential for the reproductive organs of the male and female. It strengthens the heart muscles, dilates capillary blood vessels enabling blood to flow more freely into muscle tissue.

Multi-minerals, Selenium and zinc are important. Zinc has a beneficial effect on the prostate and all the glands. It also assists the body in absorbing B-complex vitamins.

HERBAL COMBINATIONS—Blood Purifier, Bone (rich in minerals), Digestion, Energy and Fitness formulas, Glands, Immune, Lower Bowels and Stress formulas.

SINGLE HERBS—Key herbs: Damiana (tonic to glands), Ginseng (strengthens the body), Gotu Kola (brain food), Ho Shou Wu, Kelp, Sarsaparilla, Saw Palmetto. Alfalfa, Blessed Thistle, Cramp Bark, Echinacea, False Unicorn, Golden Seal.

SUPPLEMENTS—Amino Acids, Bee Pollen, Lecithin, Chlorophyll, Essential fatty acids (Salmon Oil, Evening Primrose Oil, etc.).

AVOID—Avoid hot baths and saunas which could lead to low sperm counts. Avoid smoking, alcohol, caffeine drinks. Sugar products and white flour products leach nutrients from body. Heavy metal poisoning may lead to energy loss. (Hair analysis can determine built-up metals.)

INDIGESTION
(Dyspepsia)

Indigestion is one of the most common health problems people are faced with today. If you lack hydrochloric acid and enzymes you may have bad breath, heartburn, belching and flatulence. Other problems associated with incomplete digestion are: skin problems, recurring headaches, muscle wasting, lowered immunity, delayed wound healing, anemia, poor bowel function, depression and allergies. If the food stays longer in the digestive tract than it should, constipation and diarrhea and autointoxication develops. Poor digestion is the beginning of many chronic diseases. Digestive disorders are: Constipation, Diarrhea, Acidosis and Alkalosis, Gastric Catarrh, Chronic Gastritis, Dilation of the stomach, Ulcers, Liver Disorders, Gallstones, Enteritis, Appendicitis, colitis, Diverticulosis, Hemorrhoids.

The stomach is the most abused organ of the body. Americans treat themselves with antacids, which are swallowed in unbelievable amounts each year. Along with tranquilizers and sleeping pills, antacids are the most commonly prescribed drug used today.

Antacids are not the answer. Although they offer initial relief, the stomach reacts by producing even more acid because the cause of an acid stomach has not been dealt with. Antacids slow down digestion and create flatulence. Many people use bicarbonate of soda, but it is high in salt and constant use can cause kidney stones. It also produces carbon dioxide in the stomach, resulting in belching and distension.

Hydrochloric acid is necessary for digestion and good health. It's essential for the assimilation and absorption of minerals and vitamins, as this process begins in the stomach. Hydrochloric acid also destroys many harmful bacteria, parasites, and worms that could enter the bloodstream and be carried to other parts of the body. If the bacteria and parasites and worms are not destroyed, they can set up colonies in the intestine and interfere with absorption of food nutrients.

NATURAL THERAPY—Blood Purification, Liver Cleansers and a cleansing of the entire gastrointestinal system. Juice fasts along with enemas or lower bowel cleansers. Healing and cleansing herbs to remove obstructions in the colon, stomach, liver and gallbladder. Eat only when you are hungry; avoid large meals; chew food thoroughly and with mouth closed (prevents swallowing air). Don't drink liquids with meals (hydrochloric acid is weakened).

FOODS TO HEAL—Sprouts, especially alfalfa and fenugreek, provide minerals and cleansing properties. Citrus juice such as lemons and limes in warm water are healing and cleansing for the digestive and on abnormal tissues. Combining food properly will heal and improve digestion. Don't mix proteins and starches at the same meal. A protein works well with vegetables. Starch meals work well with vegetables.

Fiber-rich foods will promote proper digestion. Whole grains, fresh fruits and vegetables, fresh papayas, pineapples and mangos are good digestive aids and provide digestive-enzymes.

VITAMINS AND MINERALS—Vitamin A, along with pantothenic acid and zinc, work together to aid absorption of nutrients in the intestinal tract. B12 needs hydrochloric acid for absorption. A deficiency can cause learning disabilities, nervousness and depression. B-complex vitamins with extra B1, B2, B6, niacinamide, choline are beneficial. Vitamin with bioflavonoids need hydrochloric acid for efficient absorption. Minerals are essential for a healthy body and manganese, calcium and other minerals need proper digestion for the body to utilize nutrients.

HERBAL COMBINATIONS—Blood Purifier, Bone formulas, Digestion, Immune, Lower Bowel, Nerve, Stress.

SINGLE HERBS—Key herbs: Bitter herbs such as Gentian and Oregon Grape are healing for digestive problems. For a nervous stomach take Chamomile tea with ginger. Acid stomach or heartburn: Raspberry tea, or one tablespoon of Slippery Elm and a capsule of Ginger in warm water. Nausea: mix together Cinnamon, Cardamon, Nutmeg, Cloves with a pinch of Ginger, in a warm cup of herbal tea. Aloe Vera juice is healing. Buchu and Capsicum, promote circulation. Comfrey is healing and will rebuild tissue. Fennel is soothing and Garlic, Gentian, great healers of the intestinal tract. Ginger, Golden Seal (great healer of the intestinal tract), Marshmallow (reduces inflammation), Papaya, Parsley, Peppermint, Slippery Elm, Psyllium. Nervine herbs: Hops, Passion Flower, Saffron (helps to digest fats), Scullcap, and Valerian.

SUPPLEMENTS—Bee Pollen, Acidophilus, Aloe Vera Juice, Glucomannan, Calcium Combination, Garlic and Peppermint Oil. Protein digestive aid, Pancreatic Enzymes.

AVOID—Antacids, alcohol, mineral oil (blocks vitamins A and B vitamins from being absorbed). Wrong food combining. Avoid eating when upset or under stress. Too much salt, sugar, spices, meat, dairy products. Chew your food very well. It has a profound effect on digestion. Avoid white rice, white bread and white sugar; they stimulate production of hydrochloric acid but cannot neutralize them. Coffee speeds up acid production. Stress inhibits gastric secretions. Antibiotics kill the bacteria flora in colon, which causes a deficiency in vitamin K and B-vitamins.

INFERTILITY

After a girl reaches puberty, now around 11 or 12 (it used to be around 16 about 50 years ago), one egg is released each month until menopause. If the egg is not fertilized by male sperm, the egg is eliminated out of the body and a new one is replaced the next month. With infertility it is obvious that something has gone wrong to either the female egg or the male sperm.

Since infertility is increasing many American couples experience unhappiness and frustration. It is now known that it is not necessarily the woman's fault, as it was thought in the past. To be barren was a disgrace, and a woman was not considered a complete person. Not so today; men are to blame in about 40 percent of the cases.

Women's problems are usually infections, venereal disease, inherited disorders, mishandled abortions, bacterial organisms, endometriosis, drugs, plugged fallopian tubes, or nutritional deficiencies. There are many more reasons, and I feel emotional trauma can be a real concern.

Birth control pills were developed about thirty years ago, and the women who have used the Pill have usually done so without fear and were convinced that it was safe and harmless.

I saw women take The Pill as eagerly as they took to the Thalidomide Drug, with confidence that since it was prescribed by their doctors it was safe and free from side effects. The Pill manufacturers are faced with hundreds of lawsuits from women who were convinced the Pill was safe. Oral contraceptives are unsafe drugs with numerous side effects. The Pill can cause permanent infertility, high blood pressure, blood clots, strokes, heart disease, kidney failure, varicose veins, and cancer of the breast, uterus and liver.

NATURAL THERAPY—Blood Purification, Lower Bowel cleansing using enemas, colonics or herbal colon cleansers. Autointoxication could be a problem. Change the diet to natural, wholesome food.

Sprouts and seeds have life-giving properties, nuts, fresh salads (using lots of leaf lettuce), cabbage, and other raw vegetables. Wheatgrass juice is an excellent food to build and clean the blood.

FOODS TO HEAL—Fresh raw fruit first thing in the morning. One half Lemon in warm water is a liver booster. Soak whole grains the night before and eat for breakfast. Make almond milk for the cereal. Carrot and beet juices are nourishing. Raw salads with lots of vegetables. Steamed vegetables. Sprouts, alfalfa, mung beans, wheat, fenugreek, radish. Eat lots of fresh fruit and berries in the season. Fish and chicken (organic). Organic eggs are nourishing. Soft boiled is nutritious.

VITAMINS AND MINERALS—Vitamin A assists in maintaining normal glandular activity and prevents sterility. B-complex vitamins protect against stress, nausea, edema, toxemia. Stabilizes female hormone levels, which is critical in conceiving. Vitamin C and bioflavonoids strengthen male sperm and female eggs. Protects against germs and viruses. Lack of this nutrient can cause varicose veins, slow healing of wounds and frequent sickness. Vitamin E is called the fertility vitamin for the male as well as the female. Lack of vitamin E is the major cause of premature babies. It helps to prevent miscarriage and increases male and female fertility. Vitamin D is essential in pregnancy to prevent rickets in infants. Multi-mineral supplementation is essential. Extra selenium, silicon, calcium, magnesium, manganese, and zinc are critical for conceiving. Kelp is high in iodine. Oatstraw is rich in silicon. Herbal calcium formula is easily assimilated.

HERBAL COMBINATIONS—Anemia, Blood Purifier, Bone formulas, Candida, Digestion, Female herbal Formula, Glands, Immune, Lower Bowels, Nerve formulas.

SINGLE HERBS—Alfalfa, Chickweed, Damiana (strengthens reproductive organs), Dandelion, Dong Quai (good for female organs), Echinacea (cleans blood), False Unicorn (helps in infertility), Ginseng (men), Kelp, Licorice, Oatstraw, Pau D'Arco, Red Clover, Red Raspberry (strengthens all female organs), Sarsaparilla (stimulates progesterone), Saw Palmetto.

SUPPLEMENTS—Acidophilus, Chlorophyll, Essential Fatty Acids, Evening Primrose oil, Safflower Oil, Salmon Oil.

AVOID—Drugs of all kinds, even aspirin (can cause birth defects). Avoid all white flour and white sugar (leaches nutrients from the body). Chlorinated water, chemicals, pesticides, herbicides. Avoid heavy metal poisoning. Check mercury and other metal poisoning in the teeth.

INSOMNIA

Insomnia is a major problem in our society today. Many have trouble falling asleep, or they suddenly wake up in the middle of the night and cannot go back to sleep. There are many reasons for insomnia. It could be anxiety, stress, lack of nutrients (especially minerals), worry, hypoglycemia, nervous tension, physical aches and pains, eating heavy meals late at night, or the brain is active late at night from stimulants such as found in cola drinks, coffee, tea and chocolate.

Insomnia is a nervous disorder, and almost all nervous disorders are affected by autointoxication. This is self-poisoning by chronic constipation. (Remember, no one thinks they are constipated, but because of our eating habits, we do not completely eliminate excess food.) The brain and the nervous system are very sensitive to toxins, and when the bloodstream isn't clean and pure, it has a negative effect on sleep.

Prescription drugs for insomnia are not the answer; they do not cure sleeplessness. Drugs do not get to the problem, they only cover the symptoms. Millions of prescription drugs are written each year for sleeping pills. They are responsible for thousands of trips to hospital emergency rooms, and many of those victims fail to leave the hospital alive.

Natural sleep is essential to restore vital energy, and give the body time to cleanse. If a person wakes up in the morning tired and exhausted it usually means the liver needs purifying and cleansing.

Research shows that people with chronic insomnia almost always have nutritional deficiencies. They usually lack the following: B-complex vitamins, Vitamin C, D, calcium, magnesium, manganese, potassium and zinc. These natural nutrients enable our sleep mechanism to function properly. We know that a lack of any B-vitamins can contribute to anxiety, depression and insomnia.

NATURAL THERAPY—Bowel cleansing using enemas, colonics or lower bowel cleanser and a diet to build up the bowels. Nervine therapy to build and strengthen the nerves. Fresh clean air will help induce natural sleep. Relaxation with natural mental therapies. Sleep in cotton garments if possible; the skin is eliminating toxins constantly and this will help skin detoxification.

FOODS TO HEAL—Whole grains, oats, millet (high in magnesium), buckwheat, wheat and barley contain B-complex vitamins. Nuts, seeds (sesame, sunflower, pumpkin), almonds (high in calcium and magnesium). Green vegetables (high in calcium). Sprouts (alfalfa, mung beans, radish, fenugreek). Kale leaves, turnip greens, mustard, spinach.

VITAMINS AND MINERALS—Multi-vitamins and extra B-complex build the nerves. Vitamin C with bioflavonoids, cleansing, and protects the nerves. Multi-mineral with extra calcium and magnesium (herbal calcium formulas are rich in calcium and minerals). Silicon, manganese, selenium and zinc.

HERBAL COMBINATIONS—Blood Purifier, Bone, Digestion, Glands, Insomnia formulas, Lower Bowels, Stress.

SINGLE HERBS—Catnip, Chamomile (tea), Hops (settles the brain), Lady's Slipper (extract), Lobelia (relaxer), Passion Flower (settles nerves), Scullcap (feeds the nerves), Valerian (helps in insomnia), Wood Betony.

SUPPLEMENTS—Chlorophyll, lecithin, Blue-green algae.

AVOID—Coffee, caffeine drinks, drugs, sleeping pills (weakens the nerves), alcohol, junk food.

LUPUS

Lupus is a chronic inflammatory disorder of the connective tissues and appears in two forms: discoid lupus erythematosus (DLE), which affects only the skin, and systemic lupus erythematosus (SLE), which generally affects other organs as well as the skin. It can be fatal and is characterized by remissions and flareups, like its cousin disease rheumatoid arthritis. There are three theories to the cause of SLE: 1. SLE is an abnormal reaction of the body to its own tissues, caused by a breakdown in the autoimmune system. 2. Certain factors may make a person more susceptible to SLE than others. Stress, streptococcal or viral infections, exposure to sunlight, immunization, and pregnancy may all affect the development of the disease. Genetic predisposition is also suspected. 3. SLE may be aggravated by certain drugs, from anticonvulsants to penicillins, sulfa drugs and oral contraceptives.

Symptoms include non-deforming arthritis (joint pain and stiffness), a "butterfly rash," and sensitivity to light. General body symptoms of SLE, may include aching, malaise, fatigue, low-grade fevers, chills, anorexia, and weight loss. Lymph node enlargement, abdominal pain, nausea, vomiting, diarrhea and constipation may also occur. Heart and kidney problems may also occur, and headaches, irritability and depression are also common.

Corticosteroids are the main medical treatment for SLE. But there are no miracle drugs. It is a complex disease. Those who use natural methods of cure have been known to be able to stop using cortisone and other drugs within six months to a year. Lupus, as well as rheumatoid arthritis, are conditions which are difficult to move out of the body. (Medical doctors and researchers believe that the degenerative diseases we are suffering from increasingly are side effects from the many immunizations people have been given over the past few decades. These immunizations have the effect of making it impossible for our immune systems to know whether a substance in the body is its own or whether it comes from the outside the body.)

Herbs, diet, and other therapies would normally help move out toxic waste matter and mucus with other problems, but not SLE. The waste simply stirs around in the bloodstream, unable to be removed from the body. This is because the body's ability to remove accumulated waste is hindered and retarded by a constant buildup of parasites. When the parasites are killed, nature has a better chance to cleanse.

Another cause is that protein molecules from dairy products (pasteurized and homogenized), can readily pass through the intestinal wall and form antigen-antibody complexes which can cause arthritis and form the complexes of SLE. (In the past it was only natural practitioners who believed this about dairy products, but this information comes from a reputable medical journal, The Journal of Allergy and Clinical Immunology.)

NATURAL THERAPY—Blood Purifiers with herbs that kill and destroy worms and parasites. Cleansing the bowels and the liver needs to be considered. A change of diet is the first consideration, for the patient should not be putting good things into his body through the front door while bringing garbage in the back. Large amounts of naturally cleansing foods like raw vegetable and fruit juices, as well as a mild food diet, are the only ways to heal this disease.

Systemic lupus is a degenerative disease whose power and final outcome depend largely upon the mental, physical, emotional and spiritual attitude of the sufferer. Never give up, for the nature of a degenerative disease is that the body is in an unnatural and confused state.

A fast of water and juices could also be used to great effect, as well as Garlic, Catnip and Cayenne enemas. Mild to moderate exercise would help. Massage of the extremities and central nervous system at regular intervals would give the body a great deal of extra support in moving toxins out.

FOODS TO HEAL—Endive, whole oats, lentils, beans, split peas, whole wheat, barley, brown rice, asparagus, green peas, sunflower seeds. Green salads, using lemon and olive oil dressing. Broccoli, cabbage, brussels sprouts, almonds, Avocados, buckwheat, millet, salmon, chickpeas, parsley, watercress; use leaf lettuce only.

VITAMINS AND MINERALS—Vitamin A (build up the immune system), B-complex with PABA. Vitamin C (essential for the connective tissues) with bioflavonoids, Vitamin E and D. Multi-minerals (essential for all healing), especially manganese, magnesium, calcium and the trace minerals, silicon, selenium and zinc.

HERBAL COMBINATIONS—Arthritis, Blood Purifier, Bone, Chelation formulas, Digestion, Immune, Lower Bowels, Nerve, Potassium.

SINGLE HERBS—The nervine herbs should be considered first. They are: Black Cohosh, Hops, Lobelia, Passion Flower, Scullcap, Valerian, Willow Bark. Black Walnut and Golden Seal (will kill parasites and worms). Garlic and Chaparral (excellent cleansers). Aloe Vera, Burdock (blood cleanser), Capsicum, Comfrey (healing to the skin and mucus membranes), Dandelion (helps the liver to detoxify), Devil's Claw (cleans deep in the cells), Echinacea (cleans blood and lymphatics), Eyebright, Fenugreek, Ginger, Hawthorn, Licorice, Lobelia, Myrrh, Oatstraw, Oregon Grape, Pau D'Arco (blood purifier), Red Clover (cleans toxins from the blood), White Oak, Yellow Dock, Yucca, Watercress.

SUPPLEMENTS—Chlorophyll, Acidophilus, Carrot and Celery juice, Chelated Cell Salts, Chinese Essential Oils (use externally for pain), Evening Primrose Oil, Fish Oil Lipids, Salmon Oil. Germanium, CoQ10.

AVOID—All white sugar and white flour products. Meat, fried food, stimulants such as alcohol, caffeine, tobacco, all drugs. Avoid sunlight. Avoid birth control pills, antibiotics: any drugs will create more toxins. Avoid too much salt.

MENIERE'S SYNDROME

(also ringing in ears, tinnitus)

Meniere's syndrome has many symptoms which could affect both ears. They are: ringing in the ears, loss of hearing, and loss of balance. Because of balance problems nausea and vomiting may occur. Acute attacks cause dizziness, nausea and vomiting. It could be so severe that one may actually keel over from the violent dizziness.

The hearing nerve is closely connected with the nerve leading from the balancing mechanism located in the innermost portion of the ear. Disturbances of the balancing mechanism, the labyrinth, may cause so much ringing in the ears that it can cause hearing impairment.

A bad diet causes plugged up ears. Mucus-forming foods can cause an accumulation of material in the head area and especially the ears. The head area requires more nutrition and circulation than any other single body organ. Poor nutrition causes clogged up tiny arteries, veins, and capillaries that help support ears and hearing. This happens over a period of years with gradual clogging up of the tubes to the ears. That's why we see so many elderly people with hearing problems. It is not only the elderly that are having hearing problems, we are seeing more and more children and even newborn babies with hearing problems. A factor causing hearing loss in our youth is noise pollution. Our ears are not meant to be exposed to loud noises for long periods of time. Nerve damage can result.

Some other causes of hearing loss are fetal damage, trauma at birth, infections, drugs (people have complained after being treated with drugs [quinine is one example]), thyroid disease, diabetes, injuries, noise exposure, or nerve deterioration and malnutrition. We have to realize that the lack of nutrients can contribute to hearing loss.

NATURAL THERAPY—Blood Purification, Lower Bowel Cleansing, and Tonification of digestive organs, nerves and kidneys. Diet change is the most important thing you can do to help change the inward health. Mucus-forming food is the cause of most hearing problems and infections in small children. This can build up throughout the years and cause other ear problems. Herbal tinctures in the ears have helped many people. This helps to get circulation in the head area, as well as supplying essential nutrients.

FOODS TO HEAL—Grape juice and green drinks are high in potassium. High potassium prevents autointoxication, a build-up of mucus in the ears. Almonds, baked potatoes with skin, apples, apricots (dried), cashews, sunflower seeds, black cherries, broccoli, carrots, dates, dried figs, leaf lettuce, lentils, dried beans, whole grains (thermos cooked).

A natural diet, high in whole grains, fresh vegetables, fruits, nuts, seeds. sprouts, legumes, beans.

VITAMINS AND MINERALS—The B-complex vitamins are very important. Extra B1, B2, and niacin are vital for balancing the body. Hypoglycemia has been connected with Meniere's syndrome. A multi-vitamin supplement with extra C with bioflavonoids, vitamin E, to carry oxygen to the head area. Multi-mineral supplement is important. One cause of fluid and pressure imbalance in the inner ear is electrolyte imbalance. All minerals especially selenium, manganese, zinc, calcium and magnesium.

HERBAL COMBINATIONS—Blood Cleanser, Hypoglycemia, Glands, Lower Bowels, Nerve formulas.

SINGLE HERBS—Key herbs: Black Cohosh, Black Walnut (sometimes parasites in the head area can cause hearing problems), Burdock, Echinacea, Garlic (in ears), Ginkgo, Gotu Kola, Hawthorn, Hops, Kelp (high in potassium and other minerals), Lady's Slipper, Licorice, Lobelia, Red Clover (blood purifier), Yellow Dock. Other beneficial herbs: Buchu, Capsicum, Chickweed, Cornsilk, Dandelion, Ginger, Ginseng, Mistletoe, Oregon Grape, Parsley, Queen of the Meadow, Sarsaparilla, Scullcap, St. Johnswort, Suma, Uva Ursi, Wood Betony, Yarrow, Yucca, Watercress.

SUPPLEMENTS—Bee Pollen, Evening Primrose Oil, Salmon Oil, Fish Oil Lipids, Blue-green algae.

AVOID—Fried foods, white flour products, and white sugar products. Smoking, alcohol, caffeine, and a high meat diet. Exposure to cigarette smoke in the household can cause chronic middle ear disease, and problems in children. Smoke is dangerous for children who have lung and nasal congestion. Ear damage increases six fold in children who grow up with passive smoke.

MENINGITIS

Meningitis is an inflammation of the membranes that cover the brain and the spinal cord, called the meninges. It is a serious disease and needs to be diagnosed and treated immediately. This is one disease that needs a doctor's attention. It was once a dreaded disease but if treated early with sulfa medicines and antibiotics can usually be cured. This is one disease that Dr. Mendelsohn has insisted that tests should be performed on.

He said, "Potential consequences of failure to diagnose and treat meningitis properly are mental retardation and death. If your child has an unexplained fever for three or four days, accompanied by drowsiness, vomiting, a shrill cry, and possibly a stiff neck, it is time to suspect meningitis. Some of these symptoms are also present with influenza. But you can distinguish meningitis by the last two, particularly the shrill cry."

NATURAL THERAPY—Prevention is the best treatment. Blood Purification. Keep the bowels open and clean. A nutritional diet using a variety of fruits and vegetables. Don't just limit a few vegetables for children, get them acquainted with all good fruit and vegetables. Meningitis is mostly common in children. When treating them for acute diseases, use natural methods to prevent a build-up of toxic material. Toxic material can accumulate in the brain area and cause diseases. Use brown rice and millet (they digest easily). Use whole grains after a baby is a year old, or has its teeth (digestion of starches depends on chewing and saliva).

FOODS TO HEAL—Fresh citrus juices: oranges, lemons, limes and grapefruit. Herbal teas, catnip, chamomile, peppermint, spearmint, red raspberry, and red clover blends will heal and help the body eliminate toxins. All green vegetables are healing. Use raw finger vegetables for children. Cut up raw and watch them eat and enjoy them: Carrots, broccoli, cucumbers, turnips, green peppers, and all raw vegetables. Children need minerals and B-complex vitamins, which are found in whole grains. Cook them in a thermos overnight: they are ready in the morning and still retain the B vitamins which are usually lost in high temperatures.

VITAMINS AND MINERALS—Vitamins A and C will help the healing process as well as prevent viruses and germs. B-complex with pantothenic acid. Multi-minerals (vomiting and high fevers lead to mineral loss). Zinc is very healing. Calcium and magnesium help protect the nerves.

HERBAL COMBINATIONS—Blood Purifier, Bone (rich in minerals), Glands, Immune, Infections formulas, Lower Bowels, Nerves, Potassium.

SINGLE HERBS—Key herbs: Black Walnut (balances minerals), Burdock (blood cleanser), Capsicum, Cascara Sagrada (cleans the bowels), Catnip (calms the nerves), Fenugreek (loosens and eliminates mucus), Golden Seal (antiseptic), Ginkgo, Gotu Kola, Hops (helps to settle nerves), Lady's Slipper, Lobelia (great nervine and clears obstruction), Psyllium (bowel cleanser), Scullcap (helps calm nerves). Other vital herbs: Aloe Vera, Black Cohosh, Buckthorn, Buchu, Comfrey, Cornsilk, Dandelion, Hawthorn, Horsetail, Ho Shou-Wu, Licorice, Myrrh, Oatstraw, Red Clover, Rose Hips, White Oak.

SUPPLEMENTS—Chlorophyll, lots of liquids. Enemas will help bring fever down quickly, liquid vitamin C, Blue-green algae.

AVOID-All white sugar products, artificial sweeteners, flavorings, and colorings. Immunizations have been linked with meningitis. This has to be up to the parents whether to vaccinate their children or not. Vaccines are full of viruses. They can remain in the body and when the immune system is low can flair up.

MENOPAUSE
(hot flashes, irritability, depression)

Menopause is the physical and emotional transition that marks the permanent cessation of menstruation, and takes approximately five years. It usually starts around the age of fifty. It can take longer if a women is in poor mental and physical health. Symptoms relating to menopause are hot flashes, night sweats, depression, dizziness, headache, difficult breathing, and heart palpitations. These have been connected with decrease in estrogen production. But if a women is in good health, assimilating nutrients and has good digestive and eliminative systems, as well as a positive outlook, these systems are hardly noticed.

With good health habits, following menopause, the ovaries continue to produce a reduced amount of estrogen. But other glands take over, the adrenals begin to form a type of female hormone which is used along with the small amount of ovarian estrogen. With the right herbs, the body can continue producing the correct amount of hormones needed by the system. Even the correct amount of progesterone is produced by other glands.

Women need to drop the amount of calories eaten, because the need is less. If it isn't decreased, there is a large chance that weight gain is inevitable. If complex carbohydrates are added to the diet, with lots of vegetables and vegetable salads and increased exercise, the body can compensate for the weight gain.

Some women start menopause early, some later. Some fertility pills can throw women into menopause way before her time. Drugs can even cause menopausal symptoms. The following drugs can cause cessation of menstruation of varying periods of time, sometimes permanently: Oral contraceptives, Busulfan, Chlorambucil, Mechlorethamine and Vincristine are used to treat some kinds of cancer. They are very strong and could cause birth defects. Cyclophosphamide is used to treat some kinds of cancer and severe cases of rheumatoid arthritis and systemic lupus erythematosus.

NATURAL THERAPY—Blood Purification, Strengthening the Glands, and Nervine Therapy. The liver needs to be strengthened and purified. The liver has the job of filtering toxins, to prevent the blood from accumulating excess hormones. Diet change is helpful in cleaning the blood and bowels.

FOODS TO HEAL—Whole grains, sesame seeds and sunflower seeds. Almonds, pecans, walnuts. Eat lots of vegetables in fresh salads and lightly steamed. Garlic, figs, dates, cabbage, broccoli, seaweeds, bananas, avocados, grapes. All fruits fresh and juiced. Foods rich in magnesium: beans, grains and dark green vegetables.

VITAMINS AND MINERALS—B-complex vitamins will help in nervous disorders especially B5 (helps in glandular function), B6 (helps in water retention), and B12 (helps in stressful situations). Vitamin C with bioflavonoids, helps in hot flashes. Vitamin E helps in all symptoms of menopause, especially hot flashes. A multi-vitamin and a multi mineral supplement should be taken with meals, they help the body to produce it own hormones. Calcium and magnesium relieves stress calms the nerves. Selenium is involved in balancing hormones. Silicon, manganese and other trace minerals help the body to utilize calcium.

HERBAL COMBINATIONS—Anemia (blood building formulas), Bone (strengthens the bones and prevents bone loss), Digestion formulas (help to assimilate nutrients), Glands, Nerve and formulas for Menopause.

SINGLE HERBS—Key herbs: Black Cohosh,(helps the body make its own hormones), Blessed Thistle, Burdock (blood cleanser), Chamomile, Damiana (help to balance hormones), Dong Quai (great for all female problems), False Unicorn, Gentian, Gotu Kola, Hawthorn, Hops, Horsetail (contains silicon for bone health), Kelp, Red Raspberry, Sarsaparilla, Squaw Vine, Saw Palmetto. Other helpful herbs: Alfalfa, Licorice, Lobelia, Parsley, Red Clover, Scullcap (strengthens the nerves), Valerian, Wood Betony, Yellow Dock.

SUPPLEMENTS—Evening Primrose Oil, Fish Oil Lipids, Salmon oil, Chlorophyll. Safflower Oil.

AVOID—Dairy products (contain antibiotics and hormones to disrupt the body's natural estrogen): milk, cream, cottage cheese, sour cream, cream cheese all contain hormones. Sugar and white four products. Avoid meat it can contribute to hot flashes. Avoid coffee, tea, alcohol, nicotine. Avoid all drugs, they disrupt the body and cause many side effects.

MENTAL ILLNESS
(manic-depressive disorder, schizophrenia)

Manic-depressive disorders cause a lot of misery for the person suffering from it, as well as their loved ones. When someone you love or someone you are acquainted with is manifesting symptoms of anti-social behavior, before you make an appointment with a psychiatrist, please examine their diet. It is loaded with artificial additives, white sugar, donuts, and pastries? Does the person smoke, drink,or consume an inordinate amount of caffeine?

Some symptoms in mental disorders are: loss of interest in school and work, changes in sleep pattern, withdrawal from society, irritability, panic attacks, sudden attacks of rage, lack of enthusiasm. Lose interest in family and friends. I met Heather in Canada and was astonished when she told me she was diagnosed as a manic depressive and a borderline schizophrenic. She was a lovely and delightful person. At age thirty she was hospitalized for a suicide attempt and her stomach was pumped. All her life she was plagued with mental problems, and her family members had the same problems. She said that desires to commit suicide and panic attacks were a way of life for her. She was on all kinds of drug therapy, using Lithium, Haldol and Oxazepan. She underwent psychiatric therapy two times a week, but nothing seemed to help.

Heather was introduced to a nutritional approach to her problem by a friend. With a complete cleansing program, using herbs to clean her blood and colon, she began to gain her sanity. She started out slowly to change her diet. She used nervine herbs such as Valerian, Lady's Slipper, Passion Flower, Scullcap, Hops, and Wood Betony. She was able to experience her first night of restful sleep. She felt her health improve immediately. She gave up her medications. Her attitude is positive, and she is now well and happy, helping others who suffer from depression.

NATURAL THERAPY—Blood Purification and Lower Bowel Cleansing. Autointoxication is the main cause of mental illness. Toxins can enter the bloodstream and to the brain and cause all kinds of disturbances. The brain and nervous system are very sensitive to toxins. A change of diet and habits are essential for mental disturbances.

FOODS TO HEAL—Whole grains, millet, buckwheat, whole wheat, barley, yellow corn meal (contain vitamin E and B-vitamins). Cold-pressed oils, beans, legumes, brown rice, Nuts (almonds, cashew), seeds, Lots of vegetables salads using dark green leafy vegetables. Use steamed vegetables, organic eggs and fish. Fruits have a cleansing effect on the body.

VITAMINS AND MINERALS—Multi-vitamin with extra vitamin E, A, and C will strengthen the nervous and immune system. B-complex vitamins (for nerves and iron absorption), extra B5 and B12. Vitamin F (essential fatty acids), promotes healing. Multi-mineral with extra calcium and magnesium, silicon, selenium and zinc. Iron (found in yellow dock) for energy and oxygen, potassium.

HERBAL COMBINATIONS—Blood Purifiers, Bone, Digestion, Lower Bowel cleansers, Gland formulas, Liver formulas, Nerves, Stress.

SINGLE HERBS—Key herbs: Black Cohosh, Blue Vervain, Catnip, Chamomile, Dandelion (liver cleanser), Hops, Horsetail (supplies silicon and calcium), Kelp (rich in minerals), Lady's Slipper, Lobelia, Passion Flower, Psyllium, Scullcap, Valerian. Other vital herbs: Alfalfa, Aloe Vera, Black Walnut, Buchu, Burdock (cleans the blood), Capsicum (provides circulation), Cascara Sagrada, Echinacea, Garlic, Gentian (heals digestive tract), Ginger, Hawthorn, Licorice, Parsley, Red Clover, Uva Ursi, Yellow Dock.

SUPPLEMENTS—Essential fatty acids (Evening Primrose Oil, Salmon Oil, Safflower Oil—cold pressed), Chlorophyll, Lecithin, Blue-green algae.

AVOID—Sugar and all sugar-containing food, animal fats, eat very little meat. Turkey, chicken and fish are best. Caffeine producers like chocolate. All refined foods.

MONONUCLEOSIS

It is called Infectious Mononucleosis and glandular fever. It is caused by the Epstein-Barr virus, a member of the herpes group. It affects mostly young adults and is rarely seen after thirty-five. It is an infectious viral disease that affects the lymph tissues and glands in the neck, groin, armpits and in the respiratory system. The symptoms are: Extreme fatigue, headaches, fever, sore throat, swelling of the glands of the neck and sometimes under the arms and in the groin. It also affects the spleen and the liver.

It is an acute infectious disease that spreads easily. Those with low immune systems suffering from improper nutrition and exhaustion are the most vulnerable. This being an acute disease, and when treated naturally will be a healing process for the body. If treated with drugs, and if a lot of heavy food is eaten, it will throw the disease into the system, solidify it and weaken the organs that are filled with toxins. This would be the glands, spleen and the liver.

This disease can be transmitted by blood transfusions and has been reported after cardiac surgery. This is a disease where the virus is in the body, and when the immune system is weakened it becomes active. This is another disease that could be the results of the mass inoculation that is pushed in our society.

NATURAL THERAPY—Bed rest is essential. Blood Purification, Lower Bowel Cleansers. Strengthen the immune system. Cleanse the body and help nature rid the toxins that are causing this disease. Citrus juices are excellent diluted with fresh pure water. Herbal teas to help nature. Red Clover blend teas and tinctures are excellent. Read the section on acute diseases to determine how vital it is to treat this disease properly.

FOODS TO HEAL—Citrus juices at first. Add fresh fruit and vegetables. Baked potatoes with skin on, Potassium broths, using potato peelings. Celery, parsley, chives, onions, cabbage and any vegetable tops. Baked squash, summer squash.

All kinds of vegetables (steamed and fresh). Use only fish, turkey or chicken. Try to get the organic grown to eliminate antibiotics and hormones. Hormones are messing up our bodies. Use only whole grains; they will restore strength and nutrition. They contain B-vitamins, minerals and enzymes (if cooked in a thermos overnight). This type of cooking should appeal to college students, because the food is ready to eat in the morning. You can even make soup broths in the thermos using brown rice.

VITAMINS AND MINERALS—Vitamin A builds the immune system and strengthens the glands. B-complex vitamins, help in stress and build up the nerves. Extra B12 will help. Vitamin C with bioflavonoids will protect the glands and immune system. It will help the healing process. Vitamin E sends oxygen to the cells and blood. Multi-mineral supplement with extra calcium and magnesium (using herbal calcium formulas). Magnesium helps counter fatigue. Potassium, silicon, selenium and zinc.

HERBAL COMBINATIONS—Bladder and Kidney formulas, Blood Purifiers, Bone, Glands, Immune and infections formulas.

SINGLE HERBS—Key herbs: Burdock, Chaparral, Dandelion (protect the liver), Echinacea (cleans the glands), Golden Seal (great for infections), Hops, Horsetail, Lobelia, Pau D'Arco (cleans the blood and protects the liver), Red Clover. Other vital herbs: Alfalfa, Black Walnut, Buchu (cleans the kidneys), Capsicum, Cedar berries, Cornsilk, Ginger, Hawthorn, Licorice, Parsley, Uva Ursi, Watercress (builds and cleans), Yarrow, Yellow Dock.

SUPPLEMENTS—Acidophilus, Liquid Chlorophyll, Essential Fatty Acids, such as Evening Primrose Oil. Cold-Pressed Safflower or Sunflower seed oil, Salmon Oil, Lysine (amino acid). A free-form amino acid supplement would be helpful. Blue-green algae is very healing.

AVOID—Chocolate, all sugar products, candy, cake, cookies, ice cream, jams, pastries. Avoid a high meat diet. Caffeine drinks. All these foods leaches out nutrients that are essential to a healthy immune and nervous system. Avoid tobacco and alcohol.

MOTION SICKNESS

Motion sickness is also called "travel sickness", and can be caused by traveling in a car, bus, boat, plane or even in a swing. It affects children as well as adults. It can result from excessive stimulation of the labyrinthine receptors of the inner ear by certain motions. The problem is created when the motion change is rapid, irregular or continuous, such as constant speed changes in a car or plane or roll of a boat. It can also be caused by confusion in the cerebellum from conflicting sensory input; visual stimulus (a moving horizon) conflicts with labyrinthine perception. Predisposing factors include tension, fear, offensive odors, or sights and sounds or evening feelings associated with a previous attack. The inner ear and the eyes contribute to the sense of balance. When these two systems send different messages to the brain it causes an imbalance. Vomiting or nausea occurs when the brain cannot figure out what to tell the body to do.

Weak muscular activity in the stomach, caused by too much congestion and mucus and fear or stress, can prevent digestion and cause a disruption. Constipation can be one cause. A weak system with weak nerves can cause motion sickness. I believe autointoxication is the main cause of motion sickness and nausea. When pregnant women have nausea and vomiting it is nature;s way of cleansing the mother's body to provide a healthy environment for the baby. When children and adults have the same problem I believe there has to be a weakness in the system, because it is not normal to have this problem.

NATURAL THERAPY—Blood Purifiers and Lower Bowel Cleansers and food and herbs to strengthen the nervous system. Nausea usually means the liver needs to be cleansed. Discourage reading, playing games or looking down when riding in a vehicle. Good posture is essential to avoid loss of energy flow to the stomach. Create good digestion and elimination. Fresh air is very important to prevent nausea and vomiting.

FOODS TO HEAL—Eat easily digested foods, until the stomach is strengthened and cleaned. Papaya juice as well as fresh. Use proper food combining to give the stomach a chance to digest foods properly. Eat a lot of steamed vegetables. Fruit is easily digested but must be eaten alone. Fresh fruit, fresh vegetables. Whole grains cooked slowly (in a thermos overnight).

VITAMINS AND MINERALS—Vitamins A and E will strengthen the mucus membranes and cells. B-complex vitamins are essential for a healthy body, they help in assimilation, digestion and elimination of food. Especially B6, which help ease nausea. Vitamin C with bioflavonoids will strengthen the stomach and help in digestion. A multi-mineral supplement is essential. Extra calcium and magnesium. Potassium is essential. Lack of it can cause incomplete digestion, constipation, nervousness and poor stomach and intestinal muscle tone.

HERBAL COMBINATIONS—Blood Purifier, Bone, Digestion, Glands, Liver, Lower Bowels, Nerve, Potassium formulas (will help stomach), Stress.

SINGLE HERBS—Ginger or Fennel tea will help settle stomach. Golden Seal and Gentian (will clean and heal the digestive tract). Lobelia extract, Hops (settle a nervous stomach), Kelp, Papaya, Peppermint tea (should always be used after vomiting), Red Clover, Red Raspberry, Scullcap, Wild Yam.

SUPPLEMENTS—Acidophilus, Alfalfa Mint tea, Chlorophyll, Green Drinks, Lemon and pure water. Blue-green algae.

AVOID—Alcohol, cola drinks, caffeine drinks, chocolate. Avoid drinking too much soda, they leach precious minerals, and vitamins from an already weakened body. Don't drink with meals. Learn to chew food well. Avoid poor food combining, so the body can restore proper digestion and assimilation.

MULTIPLE SCLEROSIS

Multiple Sclerosis is one of the most common diseases of the nervous system in the United States. It is not generally known by the public because it is not a sudden killer, and it does not usually strike dramatically. Multiple Sclerosis is a disease that affects the brain and spinal cord which comprises the central nervous system. It is a degenerative state of the nervous system due to starvation of nerves and cerebro-spinal cells.

The word Multiple comes from the damage that is produced in the many areas and sclerosis is a word that means scars. The scars that form damage the brain and spinal cord. In this disease the inflammation causes hardened patches to develop at random throughout the brain and spinal cord, interfering with nerves in these areas.

The damage is first noticed on the myelin coating around the nerve fibers. Myelin is the fatty material that acts as insulation around each nerve fiber. This leaves the nerves exposed and the impulses from the brain center run into interference as they pass through this area. The body attempts to repair itself and deposits hard material known as connective tissues (scars) which cannot conduct nerve impulses.

The exact cause of multiple sclerosis is unknown but current theories suggest that it could be a slow-acting viral infection, an autoimmune response of the nervous system or allergic response to an infectious agent. Other causes could include trauma, anoxia, toxins, nutritional deficiencies, vascular lesions, anorexia and stress. The following have been known to precede onset of multiple sclerosis: emotional stress, overwork, fatigue, pregnancy and acute respiratory infections. It is also felt that endogenous, constitutional and genetic factors may also contribute.

Symptoms include weakness, loss of bladder or bowel control, slurring of speech, tremors and blurred or double vision. Emotional disturbances are mood swings, irritability, euphoria or depression. Symptoms may be so mild that the patient may be unaware of them, or so bizarre that the person appears hysterical.

Diet intake seems to be the main factor in this disease. It is common in Canada, the United States and Northern Europe. There is strong evidence that a diet heavy in meat, sugar, and refined grains may be the main cause of Multiple sclerosis. Animal fats, those found in dairy products are links with MS. One theory is that infants feed cow's milk may be linked with nervous system disorders later in life. Breast milk has a fifth more linoleic acid than cow's milk. Linoleic acid is essential for nervous tissues.

The brain tissues of MS people have a higher saturated fat content than those without MS.

NUTRITIONAL THERAPY—Blood Purifying, Lower Bowel Cleansing. A change of diet is essential. A high-fiber and low-fat diet is very beneficial. Exercise to keep a strong circulatory system. Get plenty of sleep. Eat a balanced meal. A positive attitude about everything is essential. Correct breathing through proper exercise is important. Correct sitting is vital for proper digestion, assimilation and elimination.

FOODS TO HEAL—Fruits, vegetables, whole grains, nuts and seeds will help nourish and heal the body. Brown and wild rice. Use slowly cooked grains, steamed and raw vegetables; use raw nuts and seeds. Sprout and use them often in salads. Fish (Cod, haddock, salmon),Fruit: apples, apricots, blackberries, cherries, grapes, citrus fruit, melons, peaches, pears, pineapple, plums, raspberries, strawberries. All vegetables; broccoli, carrots, cabbage, cauliflower, celery.

VITAMINS AND MINERALS—A multi-vitamin and mineral supplement is important. Vitamin A improves resistance to respiratory infections. The following are necessary for fatty acid assimilation: Vitamin C with bioflavonoids, B6, B3 and zinc. The B-complex are very important for the nerves and especially the myelin sheath protecting the nerves. Pantothenic Acid protects the myelin sheath. Folic Acid and choline and inositol, helps in the production of lecithin. Vitamin E is vital to prevent oxidation of unsaturated fats to free radicals. Calcium and magnesium balance, potassium, phosphorus, and manganese (aids in neuromuscular control), selenium, sulphur, zinc.

HERBAL COMBINATIONS—Blood Purifier, Lower Bowel Cleanser, Digestion, Immune, Nerve, Stress formulas.

SINGLE HERBS—Key herbs: Garlic, Ginkgo (sends circulation to the brain), Hawthorn (strengthens the veins and heart), Hops (strengthens the nerves), Horsetail (builds bone, flesh and cartilage), Irish Moss (rich in minerals), Kelp, Lady's Slipper (brain and nerves), Lobelia (cleans toxins), Psyllium (food for the colon), Saffron (digest fats), Scullcap (feeds brain and nerves), Valerian (calms the nerves). Other vital herbs: Alfalfa, Black Walnut (balances minerals), Gentian (helps in digestion), Ginger, Licorice, Marshmallow, Myrrh, Oregon Grape, Slippery Elm, Suma.

SUPPLEMENTS—Essential Fatty Acids: Evening Primrose Oil, Salmon Oil, Fish Oil Lipids, Acidophilus, Lecithin (nourishes the myelin sheath around the nerves), Chlorophyll, Rice Bran Syrup (easy to digest).

AVOID—Watch for allergies, and stay away from foods that cause reactions. Dairy products, high meat diet. All sugar and white flour products. Caffeine, alcohol, chocolate. Refined foods, canned foods, white pasta products.

OBESITY

When we come to understand how harmful overweight is on our bodies, and how it can predispose us to diabetes, heart disease, strokes and many other illnesses, than we will realize how vital it is to control our eating habits. The American way of eating has given us an unhealthy appetite for damaging food. We cannot even call it food, for it doesn't even satisfy our bodies need for nutrition. If it did our appetites wouldn't be out of control.

When we start eating nutritional food, this alone will control our appetites, because our bodies will tell us, "Hey, you have given me the vitamins and minerals I need, so I won't need to beg for more". The body has a natural appestat mechanism in the brain telling when we have eaten enough, but because it has been distorted, we become obese. We have not listened to our body. We have essentially destroyed the ability of our own bodies to warn us when to stop eating. And now, because our appestat is not working properly, it is time for us to get control of ourselves and work toward losing weight.

Lack of exercise has a negative effect on appestat mechanisms. You know how our beef and poultry are fattened up? They are kept in close quarters and given hormones to make them get fatter in a shorter period, so more money can be made. Exercise promotes circulation which is an important factor in how we feel. It improves the quality of our blood. Glandular function is improved with exercise, which releases hormones necessary for health and appetite control.

Autointoxication is another reason for obesity. Our bodies are not able to eliminate each day all the waste material, and it will build up and cause overweight. We need to understand the process of digestion, which prepares nutrients for assimilation through the wall of the small intestines into the bloodstream. When we learn more about our bodies, we will become convinced that going on a diet is not the answer, the answer is to change our habits, whether it is food, exercise, or how we feel about ourselves.

NUTRITIONAL THERAPY—Blood Purification, and Lower Bowel Cleansing. Lymphatic Cleansing will also help clean the cells. It may take a year, but when the bloodstream and tissues are purified, the glands will function properly and you will see the weight come off naturally. Obesity is a chronic condition, and it may take patience and time. Chronic diseases take a long time to acquire and will take a long time to eliminate. You will feel so much better, and your whole body will feel clean and healthy. A healthy body produces a healthy mind.

FOODS TO HEAL—Fruits and vegetables. Lightly steamed vegetables will provide minerals. Fruit are cleansers of the body and vegetables are builders. Both are need in an overweight body. High fiber foods are essential. Carrot, celery, beet and apple juice are needed to feed the glands. Proper chewing, this will cut the appetite. Lemon juice in a glass of water first thing in the morning will clean the liver, which will help filter toxins. Green leafy vegetables, carrots, broccoli, celery, tomatoes, apples, cantaloupe, berries, melons, plums. Almonds, sesame seeds, seaweeds, asparagus, cabbage (red, savoy), chives. Whole grains, use thermos cooking to benefit from enzymes. Enzymes will help in proper digestion and assimilation.

VITAMINS AND MINERALS—These supplements are very important. The B-complex vitamins help to control appetite, and help in the production of hydrochloric acid. B6 works with magnesium to break down proteins, fats and carbohydrates. B12 aids the body in utilizing B6, folic acid, and vitamin C. A multi-vitamin and mineral supplement is beneficial. Vitamins A, C and E help the metabolism function better. Iron helps the thyroid (found in a balanced form in Kelp). Herbs are rich in minerals.

HERBAL COMBINATIONS—Blood Purifier, Cleansing, Digestion, Fasting formulas, Glands, Lower Bowels, Stress, Nerves, Weight Control Aid formulas.

SINGLE HERBS—Key herbs: Chickweed, Glucomannan, Burdock, Ginkgo, Ginseng, Gotu Kola, Fennel, Hawthorn, Horsetail, Psyllium, Saffron, Scullcap, Slippery Elm, Suma. Other important herbs: Alfalfa, Black Cohosh, Black Walnut (worms and parasites may be involved), Capsicum, Cascara Sagrada, Comfrey, Dandelion (cleans liver), Echinacea (cleans glands), Gentian (help in digestion), Licorice (help the adrenal glands), Marshmallow, Papaya, Parsley, Passion Flower, Sarsaparilla (helps in hormones balance), Watercress, Yellow Dock.

SUPPLEMENTS—Bee Pollen, Flaxseed, Evening Primrose Oil, Salmon Oil, Lecithin, Blue-green algae.

AVOID—All white flour and white sugar products. Chocolate, caffeine drinks. Avoid fried foods, fats and all junk food. Avoid salty food, it puts a strain on the thyroid gland.

OSTEOPOROSIS

Osteoporosis is a bone-thinning disease. It is a metabolic bone disorder which slows down the rate of bone formation and accelerates the rate of bone resorption which causes loss of bone mass. The bones affected by this disease lose essential calcium and phosphate salts and become porous like a honeycomb. They become brittle and are vulnerable to fractures even without serious falls or injuries. In fact it is usually discovered by the occurrence of spontaneous fractures of the hip,spine or long bones. It cannot be detected even with X-ray until fifty percent of the bone has been lost.

Osteoporosis is more common in women due to long-term calcium losses during pregnancies and menstruation. They also have thinner bones than men. It does occur in men, but men have heavier bones and therefore are resistant to osteoporosis, at least until their latter years.

Studies revealed by Dr. Kervran, a European scientist, found that fractures or broken bones do not knit when there are high amounts of calcium present and little or no silica present; and that bones knit extremely well when there is an abundance of silica present with little calcium. Kervran found that silica is the first most important supplement, manganese second and potassium third. Kervran feels that a significant percentage of bone breaks and fractures could be avoided altogether if sufficient silica was included daily. Horsetail and Oatstraw have high amounts of silica and manganese, copper and other nutrients.

NUTRITIONAL THERAPY—Blood Purification and Lower Bowel Cleansing will help improve digestion. A change of diet. Short fasts to improve assimilation of nutrients.

Exercise will help control bone loss. Regular exercise improves calcium absorption and stimulates bone formation. The best exercise is walking briskly, or an aerobic type exercise where you can get your heart beat up. A mini-trampoline is excellent when you use your upper body to reach your ideal heart rate.

FOODS TO HEAL—Whole grains, buckwheat and brown rice are high in magnesium and silica. Green leafy vegetables. Salads. Lightly steamed vegetables. Millet, easy to digest. Almonds, soybeans, sesame seeds, lima beans, red and white beans are high in magnesium. Sprouts will help in digestion and assimilation of essential minerals. Foods high in calcium and low phosphorus foods are: almonds, sesame seeds, kale, leafy greens, kelp, irish moss and parsley.

VITAMINS AND MINERALS—Vitamin D and C increases the absorption of calcium and other vital minerals. Fluorine, found naturally in herbs prevents bone loss. Phosphorus is vital to calcium and the ratio is important. We get too much phosphorus in meat, cola drinks and processed foods. Magnesium helps prevent calcification. It keeps calcium in solution so it can be absorbed. Half the amount of magnesium to that of calcium is needed to aid in proper calcium absorption. Silica is essential along with all minerals.

HERBAL COMBINATIONS—Bone (rich in silica), Digestion, Glands.

SINGLE HERBS—Key herbs: Alfalfa, Black Walnut (help balance minerals), Comfrey, Horsetail, Irish Moss, Kelp, Oatstraw, Red Clover, Slippery Elm. Other important herbs: Dandelion, Echinacea, Garlic, Ginger, Ginseng, Golden Seal (heals digestive tract), Hawthorn, Licorice, Lobelia, Marshmallow, Papaya, Plantain, Sarsaparilla.

SUPPLEMENTS—Evening Primrose Oil, Salmon Oil, Acidophilus, Chlorophyll, Lecithin.

AVOID—All sugar products, caffeine drinks, soft drinks, alcohol, all refined grains.

PARKINSON'S DISEASE

Parkinson's is a degenerative disease of the nervous system which is characterized by tremors and by stiffness of muscles. An imbalance of two chemicals, dopamine and acetylcholine are seen in patients, although the cause of Parkinson's Disease is not known. The chemical dopamine carries messages from one nerve cell to another and when the body cannot produce it the symptoms of Parkinsonism appear. The brain and nervous system are very sensitive to toxins and the lack of nutrients. Malnutrition is the cause of this disease in many health practitioners opinion. Another cause is the medications that older people are given. This disease occurs in later life. Some feel it may result from viral infection or carbon monoxide poisoning. I have seen dentists with Parkinsonism, when they retired and were elderly. Could mercury poisoning be one cause?

Over sixty thousand older adults develop drug-induced Parkinsonism each year. Drugs are over prescribed in excessive amounts to the elderly. The drugs most prescribed that produce this disease are for chronic anxiety and gastrointestinal complaints. Stelazine is a powerful antipsychotic tranquilizer that is prescribed to calm the intestinal tract. Doctors are not aware of this problem. It has been caught by some medical doctors when they realized what was happening. The drug Stelazine can induce Parkinsonism, then another drug is given to control the disease, when the first drug is what caused the disease.

Levodopa is one drug that is given to treat Parkinson's Disease. When levodopa is taken alone, you should avoid foods and vitamins that contain vitamin B6 (pyridoxine), since this vitamin can destroy the effectiveness of this drug. B6 is one of the vitamins that protects the system from nerve disorders. Drugs not only destroy the nervous system, they also prevent the intake of nutrients essential for brain and nerve health.

The following drugs can block the action of dopamine and cause the symptoms of Parkinson's disease: Phenothiazines, droperidol, haloperidol, reserpine (found in heart drugs, such as diupres, enduronyl, and hydropres), chlorprothixene, thiothixene, methyldopa, metoclopramide, lithium. It pays to know what drugs you are taking and what their side effects can induce.

NATURAL THERAPY—Blood Purification. Improve digestion so the nutrients can circulate to the brain. Use a natural chelation program with nutrients that dissolve toxins on the artery walls. The first natural therapy is to look for the cause, whether it is medications, heavy metal poisoning, diet or nutritional deficiencies. They need to be addressed and taken care of. Exercise is very important. A hair analysis is important to determine metal poisoning. A positive attitude is vital for improvement.

FOODS TO HEAL—Brewer's yeast, wheat germ and bran, molasses, honey, whole grains (cooked in thermos for digestion and retention of the B-complex vitamins). Whole wheat, buckwheat and millet are easily digested. Use yellow corn meal, barley, brown rice. Fresh fruit and vegetables. Use safflower and lemon juice for dressing on green salads every day. Almonds and sesame seeds are high in calcium and magnesium. Sprouts will provide nutrients that are easily digested. Eat all natural food.

VITAMINS AND MINERALS—Multi-vitamin and mineral supplements are essential. Make sure they are being assimilated. A, C, and E are vital for the immune system (along with selenium and zinc). The B-complex vitamins feed the nerves and brain (extra B6, B12, and niacin). Calcium, magnesium and silica are essential. Herbal bone combinations will provide these, as well as other essential minerals like, manganese.

HERBAL COMBINATIONS—Blood Purifier, Bone, Chelation, Digestion, Liver and Gall Bladder, Lower Bowels, Nerve and stress formulas.

SINGLE HERBS—Key herbs: Ginkgo (strengthens the brain and nervous system), Gotu Kola (rebuilds energy food for the brain), Hawthorn (for veins and heart), Hops (nerve food), Horsetail, Kelp (feeds and cleans veins), Lady's Slipper (helps tremors), Lobelia (cleanser and relaxer), Passion Flower (helps the nerves), Red Clover (cleans the blood of toxins), Scullcap (settles the brain), Suma (strengthens the whole body), Valerian (relaxer), Wood Betony (good for pain). Other vital herbs: Alfalfa, Black Cohosh, Black Walnut, Burdock, Capsicum, Chaparral, Comfrey, Echinacea, Garlic, Gentian (cleans the entire digestive system), Ginger, Ginseng, Golden Seal, Mistletoe, St. Johnswort, Yellow Dock.

SUPPLEMENTS—Chlorophyll, Lecithin, Blue-green algae. Aloe vera, Green drinks. Wheatgrass juice. Evening Primrose Oil, Salmon Oil (may help to reduce tremor).

AVOID—Avoid aluminum poisoning found in cooking pots, antacids, baking powder, pickles, relishes and some cheeses; in soft drinks and beers in uncoated aluminum cans. It is also found in anti-depressants. Avoid all drugs and stimulants; they destroy the nervous system and the brain. Caffeine, tobacco, tea, cola drinks, chocolate, high meat diet, alcohol, sugar and white flour products. They contain no nutrients and leach nutrients that are essential for the brain and nervous system such as calcium, and B-complex vitamins.

PARASITES AND WORMS

Parasites and worms are becoming a real problem in the United States. We believe our country is a highly sanitized country, but it is inside our bodies that need to be clean. The diet of the American people encourages parasites and worms. A diet rich in fat, starch and sugar provide food that these scavengers live on. A clean, well nourished body, with the production of hydrochloric acid, will provide an environment they cannot not thrive on.

One current problem that is sweeping across the country is a parasite that causes intestinal infections. It is called Giardia Lamblia, a parasite that has now become the number 1 cause of waterborne disease in the United States. Tapeworm infection is increasing by leaps and bounds. It has been linked with Americans' increasing fondness for raw and rare beef. The most deadly parasite is Amebiasis. There have even been reports of deaths from it. It is usually passed from person to person. Baiantidium parasite is from pigs and causes intestinal infections in humans. This is one main reason why pork should be left out of the diet.

Dangerous parasites are called "pathogens." The parasite which causes malarial fevers is an example of this. Many protozoans (one-celled animals) are certain type of amoeba which can destroy the intestinal lining of the of humans. They produce a painful and serious disease called "amoebic dysentery." This can cause the body to become dehydrated and eventually cause bleeding and ulceration in the bowel.

Flatworms and roundworms are parasites that can cause serious damage and can often kill their hosts. There is one type of flatworm called a "fluke" which lives and grows quite large in the intestines, liver, lungs or blood of animals and man. The tapeworm absorbs digested foods from its host, but the hookworm is the most harmful. It lives in the intestines and feeds on the blood of the host. Trichinosis is a disease from eating pork. The trichina is a tiny worm that infects pigs. The larvae, after burrowing into the intestinal wall of the pig, then enters its blood vessels. The blood carries the larvae to the muscles fiber and lives. Then when humans eat the pork, the cycle begins again in the human body. Symptoms of trichinosis are headaches, fever, sore muscles, swollen eyes, and even painful breathing. These symptoms are similar to other diseases so people do not even realize that they could have internal worms.

It was discovered that cancer may also be caused by a parasite. Dr. Virginia Livingston-Wheeler, M. D., in her book *The Conquest of Cancer*, calls the parasite the "progenitor cryptocids." This parasite begins as the lepra or tuberular bacilli and changes form to become the cancer parasite. She says that, "This microbe is present in all of our cells, and it is only our immune systems that keep it suppressed. When our immune system is weakened, either by poor diet, infected food or old age, this microbe gains a foothold and starts cancer cells growing into tumors."

NATURAL THERAPY—Blood Purification with Lower Bowel Cleansing. The body needs to be cleaned and purified. It is a wonderful machine and when nourished and treated properly will not harbor these scavengers. When there are sufficient amounts of healthy bile, the parasites and worms, their larvae and eggs, are neutralized and evacuated rapidly out of the body. The digestive system needs to be cleaned and healed. Parasites and worms cannot live in a clean body. They especially do not like minerals. Herbs have high amounts of minerals and other elements that will help eliminate them.

Sometimes people become discouraged when they try to live on a cleaner, more wholesome diet or try to go on a cleansing purge. It is hard for them to stay on it because the parasites within are crying for the kind of junk foods upon which they live and grow. It is probably wise to clean the body of the parasites first. Since the parasites cling on to the mucus in which they live the body cannot be made well even in a fasting or semi-fasting situation.

FOODS TO HEAL—Garlic is one of the best foods for pin worms. The sulphur content in garlic and onions helps to kill worms and parasites. Grind and use pumpkin seeds often on cereals they kill worms and parasites and especially beneficial for children. Grated raw beets will kill worms. Carrots (scrubbed washed and eaten with skin left on) are rich in organic minerals and sugars act as a worm killer. Figs and fig juice paralyze any worms; white figs are excellent. Papaya seeds are effective for expelling worms. Pomegranate kills worms.

VITAMINS AND MINERALS—Vitamins A, B, C, D, E, all will build up the immune system and encourage a healthy digestive system. A multi-mineral supplement containing selenium, silica and zinc discourages parasites and worms.

HERBAL COMBINATIONS—Blood Purifier, Digestion, Immune, Liver, Lower Bowels, Parasites and Worms, Potassium.

SINGLE HERBS—Key herbs: Aloe Vera, Black Walnut and Burdock (equal parts for purging out parasites and worms), Chaparral (eliminates worms), Echinacea (cleans the lymphatics), Garlic (kills worms), Golden Seal (kills worms and parasites), Horsetail (rich in minerals, discourages worms), Kelp (high in minerals, cleansing), Papaya (kills worms), Parsley (cleans kidneys), Psyllium (cleans colon), Red Clover (blood cleanser), Senna (keeps colon clean), Wormwood (kills worms), Yellow Dock (rich in iron to kill parasites and their eggs). Other beneficial herbs: Alfalfa, Buchu, Catnip, Cornsilk, Hops, Gotu Kola, Lady's Slipper, Lobelia, Pau D'Arco, Peppermint, Queen of the Meadow, St. Johnswort, Wood Betony, Yarrow.

SUPPLEMENTS—Acidophilus, Chlorophyll (cleans blood), bentonite, chelated cell salts, glucomannan, spirulina. Diatomaceous Earth. Hydrochloric acid supplements and Pancreatic Enzymes.

AVOID—A high meat diet, sugar products of all kinds. Avoid constipation, encourages worms and parasites. High fat diet.

PERIODONTAL DISEASE

According to the U.S. Public Health Service, 98 percent of all Americans fall prey to dental disease. The American Dental Association relates that by retirement time the average senior citizen has only five teeth left and 40 percent are wearing dentures.

In an advanced modern society, with the latest in technology and sophisticated knowledge, why do we as a nation have such poor dental health?

One of the first signs of dental disease is bleeding gums. When gums are inflamed, this condition is known as gingivitis. Poor diet is the major culprit in gingivitis. Lack of vitamin C can cause scurvy-like symptoms, which include bleeding gums and loose teeth. Good oral hygiene is necessary, too. Flossing daily and brushing from the base of the teeth (near the gums) toward the crown can do much to clean away plaque. Plaque, which is a film on the teeth where bacteria will flourish, can harden into a rock-like substance known as tartar. Tartar accumulates at the base of the tooth where the gum line meets. If the plaque isn't brushed off daily, the tartar irritates the gums further and causes more bleeding. The bacteria loosen the teeth from the gums and migrate lower, where they form pus pockets. This extremely dangerous condition is known as "pyorrhea". Pus will discharge into the mouth itself and the teeth actually loosen from the sockets. The roots are destroyed and so the teeth are extracted Hence, the need for dentures. This entire collection of symptoms is known as "periodontal disease". The definition of periodontal is: `of the tissues surrounding and supporting the teeth.'

Dental experts feel that loss of bone mass beneath the teeth is the major contributor to dental problems. It is called osteoporosis of the jaws. A strong bone mass is important beneath the teeth. If not it will be easier for bacteria to get in and cause further damage.

NATURAL THERAPY—Blood Purification (toxins in the blood stream can settle in the gum area). Digestion, the assimilation of nutrients vital for strong teeth and gums, need hydrochloric acid. If stomach acids are low, it contributes to poor teeth.

FOODS TO HEAL—Foods high in fluorine which strengthen teeth and bones are: Leaf lettuce, cabbage, radishes, egg whites, beets, lentils, parsnips, whole wheat, whole grains. Foods high in silicon to assist calcium assimilation: Boston and bibb lettuce, parsnip, asparagus, rice bran, onions, spinach, cucumber, strawberry, leeks, savoy cabbage, sunflower seeds, swiss chard, pumpkin, celery, cauliflower, cherry, apricot, fresh, millet, grapes, apple, sweet potato. Foods high in calcium:sesame seeds, collard and kale leaves, almonds, soybeans, mustard, spinach, filbert, chickpea, white bean, pinto beans, figs—dried, sunflower seeds, whole grains.

VITAMINS AND MINERALS—Vitamin A nourishes mucus membranes, B-complex is necessary for bones and teeth. Vitamin C with bioflavonoids prevents infections; Vitamin D works with calcium for strong bones. Vitamin E protects by enhancing oxygen to cells. All minerals are vital for bone and teeth health. Scientific research has shown how crucial silicon's function plays in calcium metabolism, bone formation, normal growth and prevention of osteoporosis and jaw bone loss. (Herbal calcium contains all minerals for bone health.) The calcium in milk cannot be assimilated properly because of the nutrients lost in pasteurizing and homogenizing. Selenium and zinc are important in healing bones.

HERBAL COMBINATIONS—Bone, Immune, Nerve, Potassium, Stress.

SINGLE HERBS—Black Walnut (strengthens teeth; brush with it), Comfrey (heals and repairs gums), Golden Seal (add black walnut and brush teeth), Horsetail (contains silica and other minerals to grow bone mass), Kelp (minerals for healthy gums and teeth), Oak Bark (heals and strengthens gums, brush teeth with it), Oat Straw, Pau D'Arco, Slippery Elm, Yellow Dock.

SUPPLEMENTS—Chlorophyll, Evening Primrose Oil, Salmon Oil, Tea Tree Oil (put some on toothpaste). CoQ10, Germanium. Hydrochloric acid and Pancreatic Enzyme supplements.

AVOID—Toothbrushes accumulate germs, rinse with alcohol to kill bacteria. Use dental floss. Avoid all sugar products, invites bacteria. Tobacco causes bone loss. Soft drinks contain phosphorus that contributes to an imbalance in calcium-phosphorus ratio. Avoid all products that will harm the immune system.

PREGNANCY

Pregnancy can be a very happy experience if the mother's body is free from toxins. Toxins can cause nausea and hormonal imbalances. Toxemia is common and a very dangerous condition for both the mother and the baby. Hormonal imbalances are due to constipation, with the liver failing to eliminate toxins faster than they accumulate. Even before becoming pregnant, parents should learn more about their bodies and the importance of a healthy diet, and the dangers of drugs, caffeine and alcohol. Even over-the-counter drugs like aspirin seem harmless, but can cause birth defects in the early months of pregnancy. Babies are being born, and die soon after or have birth defects, low birth weight, cancer, lung diseases and are addicted to drugs. Many couples planning a family are finding they have fertility problems. It is much more common now then when I was having my children.

There are many complaints of pregnancy which can be remedied naturally without resorting to drugs or over the counter remedies. Constipation, morning sickness, leg cramps, indigestion, fatigue, swollen ankles and varicose veins or backache are a few of the problems that pregnant women encounter. Pregnancy increases the bodies need for nutrients. Eating a healthy diet will provide nutrients for a healthy baby, a happy one with few demands. Also, a healthy baby has few health problems. Women on diets high in junk food have a higher incidence of difficult labors, premature babies, birth defects, infections, hemorrhages, nursing problems and problems during their pregnancy.

NATURAL THERAPY—Pregnancy is a normal function for a woman. It is essential to adopt a natural diet to provide nutrients for mother and baby alike.

A good healthy body doesn't just happen, you have to work at it. Learn the importance of food in obtaining vitamins, minerals and nutrients that assist the development of a healthy fetus. Blood Purification is essential; using herbs and green drinks will help nourish the mother and baby. Exercise will help supply oxygen for the fetus as well as strengthen the mother for easier birth. Sitz baths are common in Europe for pregnant women. In fact most bathrooms have a special sink for sitz baths. The warm or cold water brings increased circulation the pelvic area, the warm bringing increased circulation to the pelvic area and the cold water stimulated the blood to rush to that area and warm it up. It was felt that sitz baths helped almost every problem of a pregnant woman.

FOODS TO HEAL—Protein is essential, and grains, buckwheat and millet are complete proteins. A high fiber diet will keep the bowels functioning properly, as well as supply vitamins, minerals needed for mother and baby. Grains, nuts and seeds contain properties that help increase immunity to disease. Oats, yellow corn meal, barley and all grains are good. Seeds are high in calcium and other minerals, Flax, sesame, chia and pumpkin are the best. Vegetables are important, fresh and steamed. Potatoes, yams, squash, green beans can be steamed. Raw salads every day. Fruits are cleansers of the body.

VITAMINS AND MINERALS—Multi-vitamin and mineral for ideal nutrition. Vitamin A promotes growth and protects against toxins. B-complex protects the body from exhaustion and irritability. Extra B6 controls swelling and nausea. B12 creates more energy. The B vitamins strengthen the brain and heart. Vitamin C complex helps to enhance contractions and minimize stretch marks. It protects against viruses. It will protect the growing embryo from virus particles in the mother's tissues. Vitamin D is essential to help calcium absorb. It is vital for bone and teeth development and helps develop jaw bones so the teeth have room for proper growth. Vitamin E reduces the body's need for oxygen and strengthens the circulatory system and helps to prevent miscarriage. Minerals are essential; even if one mineral is lacking it could cause birth defects. Calcium is required more during pregnancy and a deficiency is caused by high meat diet. Calcium is needed with vitamin D for proper bone development. Iron builds the blood and is essential for the baby's liver. Yellow Dock contains forty percent easily assimilated iron. Silicon helps the body utilize calcium. Magnesium works with calcium. Selenium, potassium and zinc protect the immune system.

HERBAL COMBINATIONS—Blood Purifiers, Calcium or Bone formulas Immune formulas, Digestion, Lower Bowel (small doses to keep the bowels open), Nerve formulas (contain nutrients for nervous system), Stress and formulas to use the last six weeks of pregnancy for a safer and easier delivery. Some of the herbs contained in them are: Black Cohosh, Red Raspberry, Squaw Vine, Blessed Thistle, Pennyroyal, Lobelia.

SINGLE HERBS—Alfalfa contains protein and vitamin and minerals, also a blood cleanser. It is high in vitamin K which clots the blood and prevents hemorrhage. Red Raspberry tea is high in iron and calcium. Mint teas will help in nausea. Dandelion and Kelp are high in essential vitamins and minerals. Dandelion cleans and protects the liver. Kelp cleans the veins and provides nourishment. Cascara Sagrada (small amounts), Ginger (helps settle stomach), Oatstraw, Papaya, Marshmallow, Yellow Dock. Other beneficial herbs: Garlic, Hawthorn, Hops, Scullcap, Slippery Elm (rich in protein and are nourishing and healing).

SUPPLEMENTS—Acidophilus, Chlorophyll, Evening Primrose oil, Salmon Oil, Green drinks, Wheat Grass Juice, Blue-green algae.

AVOID—Alcohol (passes freely through the placenta) is very toxic to the fetus. Chemicals such as preservatives, additives, food coloring, pesticides, and any unnatural substance like MSG. Chemicals overwork the liver. Drugs should be avoided. Aspirin interferes with the clotting of blood. Antibiotics interfere with the production of RNA and protein and could cause damage to the fetus. Other problems with drugs are jaundice, respiratory problems, deformed limbs, mental retardation, digestive problems. Smoking is very harmful. The carbon monoxide prevents the intake of oxygen in the fetus and could cause birth defects and usually causes premature births. It can cause stunted growth, low birth weight and hyperactive children. Avoid sugar, white flour products and fried foods. They rob the body of nutrients.

PREMENSTRUAL SYNDROME

Premenstrual Syndrome (PMS) is not a disease but is seen as one, and it is not a mental disorder but is treated as such. Over 150 symptoms have been linked to this disorder. The most common symptoms are: Depression, irritability, faintness, restlessness, sluggishness, impatience, lethargy, delusion, indecisiveness, dizziness, nervousness, anxiety, swelling of breasts, feet swelling, constipation, hemorrhoids, skin eruptions, migraines, backaches and puffiness. The imbalance in the system could stem from genetic predisposition, an organic malfunction, a vitamin or mineral deficiency, stress, drugs or chemicals, or a combination of these. An irregular cycle often indicates the general state of a woman's health. They are usually the result of nutritional deficiencies.

Personality instability manifests itself and causes marital problems, divorce, anger, hate, bitterness and even murder. The public was stunned when a British court had reduced two murder charges to manslaughter because the accused murderers (two women), had been shown to have had "diminished responsibility" due to PMS. This is when PMS hit the news and since then has received public attention. Now women can seek help and receive it.

Some women who are accustomed to drinking alcoholic beverages often go on "binges" just before their periods. Low estrogen levels, naturally occurring during the PMS period, heighten the effect of alcohol. The drinker suffers a stronger reaction from the same amount ingested. This alleviates depression. The physical complications, related to alcohol use, are too dangerous to ignore.

Alcohol is often sought as a tranquilizer to relieve PMS discomfort. If relief is found, the results are temporary and lead to further problems.

Food cravings, unusual outbreaks of temper, and bizarre thinking affect many women within the PMS interval. Desire for sweets, or high-carbohydrate foods, caffeine drinks, chocolate, and all kinds of junk food are manifested at this time.

The liver is responsible for regulating hormonal balances. The liver is responsible for filtering blood levels of Estradiol, which is the `unfavorable' type of estrogen, and this can build up in the body. When this excess estrogen is allowed to enter the bloodstream, it travels to the brain and nervous system and causes depression and bizarre mental manifestations. Constipation is the main cause of liver being unable to filter out the excess, unwanted estrogen.

NATURAL THERAPY—Blood Purification, Lower Bowel formula, and a cleansing fast will help the liver eliminate toxins that cause PMS symptoms. The body will heal itself when given the natural nutrients. Women with severe autointoxication have very serious problems. It will take patience and endurance to implement and follow a nutritional diet to clean and build the body back to health. Nervine therapy using herbs to strengthen the nervous system is one of the best methods to help in PMS.

Physical exercise is very helpful before and during menstruation. Vigorous exercise stimulates circulation and deep breathing and improves the supply of nutrients throughout the system. Stress intensify symptoms of PMS. Stress needs to be dealt with. The mind can determine the health of the body.

FOODS TO HEAL—Food high in fiber, fruits, vegetables, grains, nuts and seeds. Brown rice and wild rice are excellent. Try cooking millet and brown rice together. Oats, whole wheat, yellow corn meal, buckwheat and millet are all high in fiber and vitamins and minerals (use thermos cooking to retain nutrients and enzymes). Yellow vegetables help keep the bowels clean. Salads, using leaf lettuce, cabbage, carrots, broccoli, and all raw vegetables are very nourishing. Also use sprouts in salads and in sandwiches. Nuts are high in protein, calcium and fiber. Almonds are the best; also use pecans, cashews, walnuts, and filberts. Grind and use seed such as chia, flax, sunflower and sesame—very high in calcium.

Foods rich in magnesium help in nerves: beans, grains and dark green vegetables.

VITAMINS AND MINERALS—Vitamin A helps to regulate the cycle and protects the glands. B-complex vitamins help combat fatigue and help to reduce sugar cravings, weight fluctuation and bloating. B-complex vitamins are vital to provide the liver material to detoxify excess estrogen in the body and prevent hormonal imbalance. B6 helps in treating tension, aggression, depression and irritability. It also acts as a natural diuretic. B2 is needed during stress. Lack of it can cause depression, hysteria, trembling and fatigue. B vitamins are needed daily. Vitamin C and bioflavonoids help strengthen the walls of the small blood vessels and the immune system. It relieves stress and acts as a natural diuretic when menstrual flow is too heavy. The C-complex has a sedative effect of aspirin, during a series of studies on rutin. Vitamin E helps ease the symptoms of PMS, relieves pain, helps in cramps, blood circulation, inhibits breast tenderness and increases resistance to stress. It is important in the production and proper metabolism of the sex hormones.

Minerals are vital. Calcium and magnesium deficiencies can cause headaches, nervous disorders, and fluid retention and pain. About ten days before menstruation calcium levels drop and remain that low until the period is over. Calcium and magnesium relieve cramps, calms and acts as a blood clotting agent. They work with vitamin D for absorption. Iodine is necessary for thyroxin to break down estrogen. Kelp is an herb high in natural iodine and other essential minerals. Selenium and zinc prevent toxins from accumulating. Potassium and silicon help regulate the body's needs, and helps in assimilation of calcium.

HERBAL COMBINATIONS—Anemia, Bone, Digestion, Female formulas, Glandular, Nerve and PMS formulas. Lower Bowel and Liver formulas will help clean the body.

SINGLE HERBS—Key herbs: Black Cohosh, Blessed Thistle, Damiana, Dong Quai (helps in all menstrual problems), False Unicorn, Hops, Kelp, Lobelia, Red Clover (cleans blood and liver), Red Raspberry (the greatest herb for all women's problems), Sarsaparilla (helps balance hormones), Scullcap (calms the nerves and brain), Squaw Vine, Saw Palmetto (balances hormones), Valerian, Wood Betony, Yellow Dock (rich in iron). Other important herbs: Alfalfa, Burdock, Chamomile (eases pain in cramps), Gentian (helps digestive system), Gotu Kola (feeds the brain), Hawthorn (circulation), Licorice (hormone balancer), Parsley (helps in water retention).

SUPPLEMENTS—Evening Primrose Oil, Salmon Oil, Spirulina, Chlorophyll, Acidophilus, Blue-green algae.

AVOID—Foods high in refined sugars and fats, highly processed foods full of chemicals. Salt causes irritability, breast tenderness and water retention. A combination of sugar and salt maximizes problems with pain and swelling.

Avoid diuretics, they cause loss of potassium and magnesium. Caffeine, leaches calcium: coffee, black tea, chocolate, and soda pop contribute to breast lumps and swelling. Nicotine destroys nutrients and produces symptoms the same as caffeine does. Alcohol destroys the liver and bloodstream.

For any problems with the reproductive system, it would be wise to avoid all food that relate to the reproductive system of animals or food that contain artificial hormones. This includes milk and all milk products which are sour cream, whipping cream, half-and half, cottage cheese, cheese. All meat of animals that have been raised on hormones, antibiotics, especially estrogen.

Chlorinated water destroys the benefits of vitamin E and causes hormone imbalance. Avoid birth control pills; they deplete the body of B-vitamins, especially folic acid, B6, and B12.

PROSTATE PROBLEMS
(prostatis, prostate hypertrophy, prostate cancer)

The prostate is a male gland about the size of a walnut and is shaped like a pyramid. It lies between the rectum and urethra. The function of the prostate is the production of the sperm cells. Life itself is a part of this gland. It is also felt that specific hormones and enzymes are manufactured there. The prostate provides a passageway for urine, and when inflammation strikes the normal flow of excretory fluids can cause pain and discomfort.

Men usually eat a lot of animal products, and this can lead to a long-term putrefaction. An autointoxication that gradually builds up in the body. The prostate is especially vulnerable to bacterial infections that seep in from toxic waste emanating from the colon. Prostatitis is inflammation of the prostate which can affect youth as well as adult men.

Prostate hypertrophy is labeled a condition of aging. It is a swelling and enlargement of the prostate usually seen in males over the age of forty. Research on prostate problems with males who suffer from this disease show their diets are usually low in fatty acids (nuts, seeds, salmon oil) and vitamin C, bioflavonoids, vitamin E and zinc.

Prostate cancer is a devastating disease that the medical doctors treat with surgery and hormone therapy. This disease is also linked to deficient diets. Cancer in women such as ovarian, breast, or uterus is also being recognized as having a connection to diets high in animal fats.

Beer and alcohol consumption in large quanities have been connected to rectal and bladder cancer. Stomach cancers are related to smoked or preserved meats, fish and chicken.

Prostate cancer, along with other diseases, first began in the twentieth century. Overly processed food has depleted vitamins and minerals from the diet. Zinc is one example. The protsate needs zinc, selenium and lecithin. A high fat diet clogs up the liver and gall bladder, and causes constipation, which eventually creates autointoxication.

NATURAL THERAPY—Blood Purification, Lower Bowel Cleansing, and sitz bath. Sit in a tub of hot water (with a horsetail infusion, put in a cloth packet to avoid mess). This can be done twenty to thirty minutes twice a day. Pure apple cider vinegar can also be used in a sitz bath. A change of diet is needed, with less meat and more vegetables, fruit, nuts, seeds.

FOODS TO HEAL—Pumpkin seeds, they contain fatty acids and are beneficial for intestinal worms. Sesame, chia and flax seeds are also high in fatty acids. Nuts, such as almonds, pine, cashew, pistachio and pecans. Whole grains (cooked in thermos), are rich in minerals and B vitamins. Green salads containing sprouts, parsley and watercress are beneficial. Steamed vegetable such as winter squash, carrots, asparagus, broccoli, cabbage are high in minerals.

Dried beans, endive, hazelnuts, dried peas, brown rice, soy flour, cashew, brazil nuts, corn, and sunflower seeds are all high in magnesium, which helps prevent infections.

Water is very important; about eight glasses a day. This dilutes urine to help avoid bacterial growth in the bladder and helps "flush" the prostate urethra.

VITAMINS AND MINERALS—Vitamin A and E are both a protection against infections. Nutritionists have found vitamin C very effective in correcting prostate infections. Large amounts are needed. Used with bioflavonoids, they work together. A multi-mineral supplement is vital to help to avoid infections. Especially magnesium, potassium, silicon and zinc.

HERBAL COMBINATIONS—Blood Purifer, Chelation, Glands, Immune formulas. Infection, Kidney, Lower Bowels, Pain (when present), Prostate formulas.

SINGLE HERBS—Key herbs: Alfalfa, Buchu, Comfrey, Cornsilk, Damiana, Garlic, Ginseng, Golden Seal, Horsetail, Juniper Berries, Kelp, Parsley, Red Clover, Saw Palmetto (helps to shrink prostate to relieve pain), Uva Ursi. Other beneficial herbs: Black Cohosh, Black Walnut, Blessed Thistle, Burdock, Chaparral, Capsicum, Dandelion, Echinacea, False Unicorn, Ginger, Hawthorn, Hops, Lady's Slipper, Marshmallow, Pau D'Arco (blood purifier), Red Clover, St. Johnswort, Wood Betony, Yarrow, Yellow Dock.

SUPPLEMENTS—Bee Pollen (good for prostatitis), Essential Fatty Acids (Safflower, sunflower, oilve oils), Evening Primrose Oil, Salmon Oil, Chlorophyll, Lecithin (assists in functions of the EFA, also dissolves fats to prevent cholesterol). Royal Jelly is good. Germanium and CoQ10 are beneficial for circulation.

AVOID—Alcohol, caffeine and nicotine have a negative effect on the prostate. Avoid a high fat diet, especially fried foods (they create free radicals, which destroy cells). Coffee is bad, even decaf because the aromatic oils cause the trouble. Once the prostate becomes enlarges or even slightly irritated it becomes very susceptible to the effects of alcohol, strong coffee, tea, uric acid in meat and drugs.

RAYNAUD'S DISEASE

(poor circulation to the hands and feet)

This is a disease of the small arteries. It affects the circulatory system. There is interference with the supply of circulation to the fingers and toes. They become very sensitive to cold. After exposure to stress or cold, the skin of the fingers changes colors from blanched, to blue or red. Numbness and tingling may also occur. These symptoms can be relieved by warmth.

This disease was first discovered and explained by a Frenchman one hundred years ago when he described a tightening of the arteries extending to the hands and feet. When they become cold there is less blood sent to the skin, and so the outlying arteries contract accordingly.

Some drugs that affect the blood vessels such as antihypertensives and channel blockers can also cause this disease.

NATURAL THERAPY—Blood Purification, and Circulatory Therapy. Keep the hands and feet warm at all times amd avoid injury to them. Change of diet, adding raw vegetables amd eating less fatty, fried foods, and meat. Add as much natural food to the diet as possible.

FOODS TO HEAL—A high fiber diet, using whole grains, freshly ground to retain all the nutrients. All the ingredients in grains work together to prevent diseases. Millet, Buckwheat, barley, whole wheat and rye are all good grains. Beans, and lentils are very good. Use sprouts in salads. Fresh and steamed vegetables. Lots of fresh fruit. Nuts and seeds.

VITAMINS AND MINERALS—Vitamin E is very important to improve circulation. Vitamin B-complex is important for liver health in the metabolism of fat. Niacin improves circulation by dilating the small arteries. Vitamin C with bioflavonoids will help strengthen and clean the small arteries.

HERBAL COMBINATIONS—Blood Purifiers, Chelation, Digestion, Heart, Potassium, Stress formulas.

SINGLE HERBS—Key herbs: Butcher's Broom (improves circulation and strengthens the veins), Capsicum (cleans veins), Garlic, Ginkgo (improves circulation), Hawthorn (strengthens the arteries and heart), Ephedra, Ginger, Ginseng, Gout Kola, Horsetail, Parsley, Saffron, Scullcap. Other important herbs: Black Cohosh, Bugleweed, Blessed Thistle, Burdock, Cramp Bark, Dandelion, Lobelia, Mistletoe, Oatstraw, Passion Flower, Rose Hips, Yarrow.

SUPPLEMENTS—Chlorophyll (strengthens veins and arteries), Lecithin (prevents fatty deposits), Essential Fatty Acids, Evening Primrose Oil, Salmon Oil, Safflower and Sunflower Oils. Glucomannan, Germanium and CoQ10.

AVOID—Injury to hands and feet. If the disease is severe maybe a warm climate would be best. Avoid all food and beverages that would interfere with health and good circulation: Alcohol, coffee, tea, colas drinks. Avoid sugar, it robs vital nutrients necessary for good circulation. Avoid certain drugs that interfere with the body's natural healing process.

RHEUMATIC FEVER

Millions of people are treated annually for strep infections to prevent Rheumatic Fever, a disease that rarely exists anymore. The risk of the treatment for this disease, penicillin, is more of a health hazard than the disease. The one risk of this disease is with the families living in poverty and unsanitary conditions. Studies have shown that rheumatic fever is related to the density of children per room. Fresh air, good nutrition, and clean sanitation are lacking and seem to go hand in hand with this disease.

Rheumatic Fever is caused from a streptococcal bacteria, causing infection with strep throat, tosillitis, scarlet fever or ear infection. If left untreated, it can affect the heart, brain and joints. It can be a serious disease, but in most cases these symptoms can be treated naturally with antibiotic herbs. It is very seldom that children get this disease.

Symptoms resembling arthritis are caused by disorder of the connective tissues. The symptoms are pain, inflammation, stiffness, joint pain and fever. Skin rash has also been seen. After the body has been weakened with rheumatic fever it can occur again.

If rheumatic fever does occur, in my opinion, it is better to use the antibiotics to clear up the infection, and then clean and purify the body of the drugs and toxins after it is over. This way you can avoid permanent kidney or heart damage.

NATURAL THERAPY—Blood Purification, Lower Bowel Cleansing, Juice fasting, enemas, using garlic/catnip. While the acute symptoms last, use only fresh citrus juices and herbal teas (red raspberry, peppermint, catnip) to assist the body in healing. Use herbal extracts that will assimilate into the bloodstream for a speedy recovery.

FOODS TO HEAL—These foods will help keep the body clean and prevent such serious infections: Ground seeds, sesame, sunflower, and pumpkin. Brown rice and millet (thermos cooking): They are less mucus forming. Vegetables such as carrots, sweet potatoes, parsley, sprouts, turnips broccoli, brussels sprouts, cauliflower, winter squash, cabbage, onions. Fruit is cleansing: use apricots, citrus fruits, apples, berries, and grapes.

VITAMINS AND MINERALS—Vitamin A is a protection to the mucus membranes and prevents harm from germs and viruses. Vitamin B-complex is needed for healing and building the immune system. Vitamin C with bioflavonoids helps eliminate infection, pain, and flushing toxins in the body.

This vitamin works with A for healing and absorption of calcium and minerals. Vitamin E provides oxygen for cell cleansing and health. Multi-minerals are important, for all minerals are need for healing (liquid for fast assimilation). Extra calcium, magnesium, potassium selenium, silicon and zinc.

HERBAL COMBINATIONS—Blood Purifiers, Bone formulas, Colds and Flu, Immune, Pain and Stress formulas.

SINGLE HERBS—Key herbs: Alfalfa and mint teas (hot), Catnip, Chamomile (soothing and calming), Cascara Sagrada (open the bowels), Echinacea (clean the lymphatics), Garlic (natural antibiotic), Ginger (baths are good), Golden Seal (relieves itching and a natural antibiotic), Hops (relaxing for the nerves), Pau D'Arco (cleans and protects the liver), Peppermint (settles the stomach and helps the body eliminate toxins), Pleurisy Root (helps in the pain), Red Raspberry, Scullcap. Other important herbs are: Capsicum, Eyebright, Lady's Slipper, Lobelia, Mullein, Red Clover, Rose Hips, Saffron, Yarrow, Yellow Dock.

SUPPLEMENTS—Chlorophyll, Essential Fatty Acids, Evening Primrose Oil, Salmon Oil, Safflower, Sunflower Seed, and Olive oil (cold pressed). Instant vitamin and minerals.

AVOID—Stop eating, the stomach is accumulating the toxins squeezed out of the cells. The acute disease is a cleansing and healing of the body. If normal eating is continued this stops the natural cleansing and healing process. This will cause the rheumatic fever to recur or cause damage to organs of the body. Avoid all sugar products. They deplete vital nutrients from the body. To avoid these diseases stay away from all white flour products, white rice, refined grains, potato chips, fried foods, bacon, sausage, ham, smoked meat and fish, hot dogs, salami, bologna, cold cuts, corned beef, chocolate, cafffeine drinks, cola drinks. All food with preservatives and additives.

SENILITY

Senility seems to go along with aging. It is called feebleness of mind and body associated with old age. Drugs are one of the main causes of memory loss or senility along with lack of nutrients. Older people are over prescribed with drugs that are given in larger amounts than their body can excrete. They are given tranquilizers, high blood pressure drugs; all kinds of drugs for nervous system diseases. This affects the brain and nervous system. When drugs are prescribed it is felt by many health doctors that they should be given in smaller amounts and less frequently. They feel our elderly are being drugged into senility.

The brain is our most sensitive organ and reacts to poor nutrition, drugs, air pollution, and bad water. When a brain neuron dies it can never be replaced. The brain is vulnerable to lack of oxygen or glucose. It can be destroyed by drugs, alcohol and drugs together, concussion, stroke and inflammation. Malnutrition during gestation and in early childhood causes irreparable damage to the structure of the brain. Alzheimer's disease shows a loss of memory and autopsies on those individuals disclosed extremely low brain levels of biochemical raw material essential for synthesizing neurotransmitters which help make remembering and thinking possible. The lack of nutrients to the brain can cause serious problems with our memory. Hypothyroidism and hypoglycemia can cause memory problems and distorted thinking.

NATURAL THERAPY—Blood Purification, Liver and Kidney cleanse (toxins in the liver and kidneys are suspected as one cause). Autointoxication is another cause of memory loss and senility. Cleansing the bowels with enemas, colonics or lower bowel formulas will help. A change of diet; the elderly are not getting enough nutrients. They usually lack B-vitamins, vitamin E, C, and minerals. Calcium is lacking along with hydrochloric acid to help in assimilation of calcium.

An hair analysis can determine heavy metal poisoning as well as a lack of vital minerals.

FOODS TO HEAL—Most food intake should be raw or slow cooked to retain all nutrients. Seeds, whole grain, raw nuts, homemade yogurt. Brown rice, millet, buckwheat, wild rice. Eat plenty of fiber food. Use psyllium hulls to keep the colon clean. Fresh fruit and vegetable salads provide enzymes for assimilation. Fish is good for memory, eggs (organic) and soft boiled. Foods high in nucleic acid containing DNA and RNA are salmon, sardines, oysters, soybeans, wheat germ and lentils. Bee Pollen and Spirulin also contain DNA and RNA.

VITAMIN AND MINERALS—Lack of B-complex vitamins, especially B1, are symptoms of a bad memory as well as lack of energy. B12 is involved with memory problems, depression and nervous system disorders. All the B vitamins work together. Vitamin A protects the immune system and is involved in keeping the mucus membranes, eyes, skin all healthy. Vitamin C with bioflavonoids help keep the arteries, and veins and capillaries healthy and clean. Vitamin E helps improve circulation to the brain. Multi-minerals are vital for health. Calcium and magnesium, potassium, (use herbal formulas for proper assimilation of calcium), silicon, selenium (detoxifies heavy metals, drugs and herbicides and pesticides), and zinc. Minerals help in detoxification of heavy metals.

HERBAL COMBINATIONS—Bladder and Kidney formulas, Blood Purifer (use red clover blend teas or formulas), Chelation, Digestion, Glands, Immune, Liver and Gall bladder and Lower Bowel formulas.

SINGLE HERBS—Key herbs: Dandelion (liver health), Echinacea (cleans the lymphatics), Garlic, Gentian (keeps digestive system clean), Ginkgo, Ginseng, Gotu Kola (food for the brain), Hawthorn (food for the heart and brain), Hops (nourishes the nerves and brain), Kelp, Pau D'Arco (great for blood and liver), Prickly Ash (circulation problems), Red Clover, Scullcap (cleans the veins and protects nerves), Suma. Other important herbs: Alfalfa, Black Cohosh, Black Walnut (parasites and worms), Capsicum (great for circulation), Oregon Grape, Yellow Dock, Yucca.

SUPPLEMENTS—Chlorophyll and green drinks. Lecithin (contains choline which is important for healthy brain cells). Germanium and CoQ10 both important for circulation and brain function. Blue-green algae for clean veins, so pure blood can reach the brain.

AVOID—Avoid stress, it can lead to loss of nutrients to the brain cells. You can learn to control stress and enjoy life. Avoid alcohol, caffeine, tobbaco, fried foods, too much meat. Eat more fish. Avoid all products that contain alumnium or other heavy metals. Avoid a high fat diet, it can clog up capillaries and arteries leading to the brain. Too much sugar and salt can contribute to the production of free radicals and loss of vital nutrients for brain health.

SEXUALLY TRANSMITTED DISEASES
(venereal disease)

Venereal disease is usually transmitted as a result of imtimate contact through sexual intercourse. Syphilis and gonorrhoea are the two most common types of sexually transmitted diseases. Chylamydial is another venereal disease that is occurring in epidemic proportions. It creates urinary tract problems in women and prostatic inflammation in men. It can cause sterility in women. These diseases are not going away, and medical treatment has not prevented the spread of these serious diseases by using anitbiotics and other treatments.

The "new sexual morality" has been sweeping the country for many years now, but people are thinking twice about loose morals with the mordern day plague AIDS spreading like a wild fire. Other sexually transmitted diseases are: chancroid, venerecum, granuloma, inguinal, genital herpes, chlamydia, trichomoniasis and AIDS.

These disease cause untold misery. Depending on the type of venereal disease the following are symptoms: painful urination, acute inflammation in the pelvic area, vaginal discharge, abnormal menstrual bleeding, brain damage (syphilis), damage to the spinal cord, heart, liver, blood vessels or other vital organs of the body. Syphilis can cause insanity, paralysis, and death, if not treated in time. If a pregnant woman has a venereal disease there is a pretty good chance her baby will be affected. This could mean birth defects, death, blindness, heart trouble, or other health problems.

These diseases used to be treated with mercurial compounds; now they are usually treated with penicilin and other antibiotics. These diseases are acute, and the body tries to clean and purify, but when they are supressed by drugs they are thrown deeper into the system to cause problems later. These are serious diseases, and probably need drugs, but after the treatment, effort must be made to clean the body as well as the drugs from the system.

NATURAL THERAPY—Germs and viruses will not attack a clean body. Work to keep the body clean both inside and out. Early treatment is necessary to prevent tissue damage. Afflicted persons should abstain from sexual intercourse and intimacy to prevent spreading the disease. Blood Purification should be started along with Lower Bowel Cleansing. If drugs are necessary, add acidophilus to prevent candida. Sitz baths will help ease pain and heal. Use herbs to help healing: Pau D'Arco, Chaparral, Red Clover and Black Walnut in sitz bath will help the healing. Use short fasts to clean the body of the impurities. There are also external Golden Seal salves that will speed the healing.

FOODS TO HEAL—Fruit will cleanse and purify the body: Cherries, grapes, plums, black currants, berries, papaya, lemons, limes, oranges and grapefruit. Eat the white of the citrus fruits: it is very healing. Vegetables are building, they contain a lot of minerals: green peppers, parsley, broccoli, Brussels sprouts, cauliflower, red cabbage, chives, spinach, sprouts, turnips.

Protein is needed for tissue repair. Use almonds, sesame, chia, sunflower and pumpkin seeds. Millet and buckwheat contain protein and are easy to digest. Use a lot of fruit juices for healing and cleansing the body. Protein drinks will help the healing process.

VITAMINS AND MINERALS—High doses of vitamin A and C with bioflavonoids are very healing. Vitamins K and E will also help the blood and provide oxygen to the cells. Multi-mineral with extra silicon, selenium and zinc. Calcium and magnesium, manganese, potassium are also needed to help balance the pH factor in the body.

HERBAL COMBINATIONS—Blood Purifiers, Candida, Immune, Infection formulas, Lower Bowels, Parasites and Worm formulas, Stress and a Bentonite Cleanse will help.

SINGLE HERBS—Key herbs: Black Walnut, Burdock, Chaparral, Echinacea, Garlic, Gentian, Golden Seal, Kelp, Oatstraw, Pau D'Arco, Red Clover, White Oak, Yellow Dock. Other helpful herbs: Alfalfa (contains vitamin K), Buchu (cleans kidneys of impurities), Capsicum, Comfrey (tissue repair), Fenugreek (help clean the mucus membranes), Hawthorn (protects the heart), Horsetail (rich in silicon for healing), Red Raspberry, Slippery Elm (rich in protein for healing), Uva Ursi (cleans the kidneys), Yarrow.

SUPPLEMENTS—Acidophilus, Chlorophyll, Black Walnut extract (use internally and externally), Salmon Oil, Evening Primrose Oil, Golden Seal extract. Tea Tree Oil (external), Blue-green algae (help purify the blood).

AVOID—All sugar products, candy, ice cream, cakes, pies, pastries. Also avoid all white flour products. They leach out the minerals that are necessary for healing. Avoid alcohol, tobacco, tea, coffee and chocolate.

SHINGLES

(herpes zoster)

Shingles is a disease that affects the nerve endings in the skin. It is the same virus that causes chicken pox, and can occur in adults who had chicken pox as children. It is felt by some medical scientists that after one is exposed to the chicken pox virus, it lies dormant in an individual's body until it may be reactivated decades later in the form of shingles. It is characterized by blister and crust formations as well as severe pain along the involved nerve. This could last for several weeks. It usually occurs on the chest and abdomen,but may occur on the face, around the eyes, on the forehead, neck and even the limbs and hands. The blisters will become crusty scabs and drop off. The elderly may suffer from attacks of shingles even after the healing takes place. The pain may continue for months after the symptoms disappear.

This is a virus that can lay dormant in the nerve ganglia and spinal cord for years until the immune system breaks down. This, in my opinion, can be caused from vaccinations or from drugs used to supress diseases. Shingles is an acute disease; a healing and cleansing of the body. When this disease is supressed it is pushed deeper into the system to cause even more serious problems. If this disease is treated naturally it will only clean and heal the body.

NATURAL THERAPY—With natural treatments of diseases you can start from the first appearance of the symptoms; you don't have to wait for days, and numerous tests to find out what the disease is first. Fasting is the first law of nature to use with an acute disease. When eating during an acute disease, the body has to stop and use its energy to digest the food rather than use it to eliminate the toxins. Use Blood Purification along with Lower Bowel and Kidney formulas. Use citrus juices, herbal teas and herbs to help nature do its job.

The skin is called the third kidney. When the kidneys are plugged up, (its like a filter that gets thick with mucus) then the skin has to take over. This is why the skin breaks out; it is trying to help the kidneys.

FOODS TO HEAL—Citrus juices are cleansing. Herbal teas will help nature do its job: Chamomile calms the nerves, Alfalfa mint will help the stomach do its cleansing job, Red Clover Blend tea will help clean the blood and Pau D'Arco will clean the blood and protect the liver. When the healing has taken place with juices and fasting, you can add vegetable broths, vegetables (steamed at first) and then raw salads and vegetables.

Make a paste with Aloe Vera Juice, Black Walnut, Comfrey and powdered vitamin C. This will help the itching and speed healing.

VITAMINS AND MINERALS—Massive doses of Vitamin C will help speed the healing; use with bioflavonoids for better results. The vitamin C increases the activity of lymphocytes and improves the migration and mobility of leukocytes, which help the immune system. Some have taken 10,000 mg. a day to start with. Vitamin A will speed the healing of the rash. Calcium is necessary to assure assimilation of Vitamins A, D and C. Vitamin E provides oxygen to the cells. B-complex vitamins are healing (use extra B12 and B1 until the symptoms disappear). A multi-mineral is very healing, with extra calcium and magnesium, potassium, manganese, silicon, selenium and zinc. A cream made with zinc will speed healing of the eruptions.

HERBAL COMBINATIONS—Blood Purifier, Digestion, Immune, Lower Bowels, Kidney and Bladder, Nerves and Stress formulas.

SINGLE HERBS—Key herbs: Aloe Vera (internally and externally), Black Walnut (heals skin eruptions), Blue Vervain, Comfrey, Dandelion (helps the liver eliminate toxins), Echinacea (helps the lymphatics to eliminate toxins), Garlic (natural antibiotic), Kelp, Lady's Slipper (excellent for the nerve endings), Red Clover, Scullcap, Wood Betony, Yellow Dock. Other important herbs: The nervine herbs are good: Black Cohosh, Hops, Chamomile, Passion Flower, Valerian.

SUPPLEMENTS—Use lysine with vitamin C, Cystine (detoxifies toxins). Good free-form amino acids are beneficial. Chlorophyll, Rice Bran Syrup, Chinese Essential oils (rub on blisters), Essential Fatty Acids, Salmon Oil, Evening Primrose Oil, Safflower or Olive Oil (cold pressed only). Blue-green algae.

AVOID—Stop eating solid foods for the first three days to help nature cleanse. Avoid all sweet fruits, white sugar products, caffeine drinks, alcohol, white flour products. White rice, pastries, sugar substitutes, and all food (junk) that will interfere with the cleansing and healing process.

Avoid stress; take long walks in the fresh air and learn to radiate a positive attitude with tolerance and love.

SINUSITIS
(sinus infection)

Sinusitis is an inflammation of one or more of the sinus cavities, or passages. Acute sinusitis is usually caused by colds or bacterial and viral infections of the upper respiratory tract, nose or throat.It occurs in the nasal sinuses, which are located in the bones surrounding the eyes and nose. Injury to the nasal bones, irritants such as fumes, air pollution, smoking and growths in the nose can cause chronic sinusitis.

An over-acid condition in the stomach will cause sinus infections. Infections are suspected if the mucus drainage is greenish or yellowish. Poor digestion of starch, sugar and dairy products will cause a runny nose. Too much of one food and eating to excess can also cause sinus infections. Allergies can cause an infection. If the drainage is clear and continues after a cold is gone, it usually means it is an allergy.

A typical sinus headache usually begins in the face, under the cheekbones often near the eyes. Sinusitis is usually caused by a cold, flu, measles, sore throat, infected tonsils, decayed teeth, enlarged and infected adenoids, cigarette smoke, and dusty air. Vitamin deficiencies can be a cause. Vitamin A is essential for the health of the mucus membranes. Symptoms of sinusitis include facial pain, earache, headache, toothache, tenderness on the cheekbones, face and forehead.

The sinuses drain down the throat, and if there is infection it can affect the lungs, and cause asthma, bronchitis, laryngitis, or even pneumonia.

NATURAL THERAPY—Sinusitis is an acute disease that needs to be treated naturally to prevent it from developing into a chronic condition. Blood Purification, Lower Bowel Cleansing, a cleansing of the mucus membranes of the stomach are necessary for clearing up of sinus infections. A change of diet, eliminating mucus forming foods and introducing raw nourishing whole foods will help. Fasting and using herbs will help dissolve hardened mucus that has accumulated in the sinuses for years. A tea made of Golden Seal and Fenugreek and snuffed up the nose will help heal infections. The Fenugreek will loosen the material and the Golden Seal will heal. Fenugreek tea taken internally over a period of time will clean mucus from the body.Also use a hot water vapor steam bath, using essential Chinese oils to make the sinuses feel better.

With sinus problems a heavy breakfast in the morning is a mistake. In the morning the mucus linings and tubes in the sinus cavities are relaxed and in a cleansing state and need time and nutrients for healing the mucus linings.

In 1909 Dr. J. A. Stucky, M.D. wrote an article in the *Journal of the American Medical Association*, addressing Intestinal Autointoxication and conditions of the Ear, Nose and Throat. He said, "Unsatisfactory results obtained after months of surgical and local treatment of some diseases of the ear, nose and throat have stimulated a more careful search for reasons why permanent relief was so rarely obtained. The question of intestinal autointoxication has at last come to the front where it belongs and has gained wide attention from the medical profession, both in Europe and America and the results and treatment of putrefaction and toxemia originating in the intestinal canal have become matters of great importance." "We know that when the middle ear and nasal accessory sinuses suffer from "air hunger" as a result of imperfect or obstructed drainage and ventilation they do not function normally. Retained secretions become purulent (discharging pus), and lead to sepsis (poisoning caused by the absorption into the blood) and various functional disturbances: gastric, neurotic, circulatory and mental."

FOODS TO HEAL—Juices (carrot and celery), green drinks, using pure apple juice or pineapple juice with parsley, watercress, carrot and celery tops, comfrey, chives and other greens. For acute attacks, stop eating and use juices from lemons, limes, oranges or grapefruit. Pure water to help flush out toxins. Fruit juices are cleansing and vegetable juices are healing. A lot of steamed vegetables and raw vegetable salads. Fresh fruit should be eaten in the morning, to help nature clean the mucus membranes.

VITAMINS AND MINERALS—Lots of vitamin A during an acute attack up to 1000,00 I.U.). Vitamin B-complex with extra pantothenic acid. Vitamin C with bioflavonoids for healing and repairing diseased mucus membranes. Multi-mineral tablets are healing. Calcium and magnesium, potassium, manganese, selenium, silicon, and zinc.

HERBAL COMBINATIONS—Allergy (usually contains ephedra for swelling), Blood Purifiers, Candida, Immune and Infections formulas, Lower Bowels, Digestion (for assimilation), Lung and Pain formulas.

SINGLE HERBS—Key herbs: Aloe Vera (healing), Ephedra, Burdock, Capsicum, Comfrey (repairs tissues), Echinacea (for infections), Fenugreek (dissolves mucus), Garlic (antibiotic), Ginger, Golden Seal (antibiotic properties), Lobelia, Marshmallow, Mullein, Pau D'Arco, Red Clover, Rose Hips, Slippery Elm (healing and provides protein for tissue repair), White Oak, Yellow Dock.

SUPPLEMENTS—Bee Pollen, Chlorophyll. Evening Primrose Oil, Salmon Oil, Olive Oil, Blue-green algae.

AVOID—Mucus-forming foods: milk, cheese, meat, too many starches, sugar, salt, and pastries. Sinus medications: they stop the cleansing process.

SKIN PROBLEMS
(Eczema, Dermatitis, Psoriasis)

The skin has a very vital function in eliminating toxins, gases, pollution and vapor from the system. Two quarts of these toxins are released every day if the pores are clean and free from build-up dead cells. If the skin is closed because of dead cell build-up, these toxins are thrown back into the body for the other organs of elimination to take over.

When the body has enough energy and vitality and the blood is clean, the channels of elimination will take care of the toxins of vapor, gases and water which were not eliminated from the skin. But if the body is overloaded with waste and toxic material, and if the bowels and kidneys are already weakened through continued over work and over-stimulation, along with toxic blood and low vitality, this is when nature causes an acute disease to manifest itself. This is when the body says, "we are going to cause a natural elimination to get rid of the waste and poisons causing low vitality in the body."

When the body is loaded with toxins, and is exposed to drafts, cold, and wet weather, the toxic matter is thrown into the circulation. When the skin is chilled, the pores are closed and it causes the blood to recede into the internal organs and as a result the elimination of poisonous gases, vapors and toxins are suppressed. If the other normal channels of elimination are also shut down then the toxins are thrown into the mucus linings and cause irritation to the nasal passages, throat, bronchi, stomach, lungs or the genitourinary organs. This produces the symptoms of inflammation, infections and catarrhal elimination, sneezing, coughs, runny nose, diarrhea, leucorrhea , etc.

Skin diseases are a sign of toxic irritation. When the skin is not properly cleansed the dead cells, rancid oil, perspiration, wastes, bacteria that accumulates and causes blackheads, pimples, whiteheads on the clogged pores. A film of dirt and pollution, accumulates daily on the surface of the skin. When the body is overloaded with mucus and fat deposits, the kidney, liver and digestive organs cannot process and eliminate fast enough and therefore the body expels through the skin.

NATURAL THERAPY—Blood Purification, Lower Bowel Cleansing. The liver and kidneys need to be cleaned of impurities. Skin brushing will help keep the skin clean so its pores can eliminate excess toxins. Juice fasting will help keep the blood clean. Exercise is beneficial for lymphatic cleansing, and the elimination of toxins.

The skin needs skin brushing, massage, fresh air, exercise, sunlight and hot and cold showers.

FOODS TO HEAL—Carrots and carrot juice. Apricots, Kale, Mustard spinach, collard greens, parsley, turnip greens, mustard greens, cabbage, chives, watercress, sweet red pepper and green peppers, winter squash are all high in vitamin A. Fruit is healing and steamed vegetables are high in minerals. Eat lots of green salads. Brown rice (cooked in thermos) will retain nutrients for healing the skin. Millet is easily assimilated.

VITAMINS AND MINERALS—Vitamin A is needed for skin health. B-complex with extra B2, B6 and niacin is helpful. Vitamin D works with vitamin a for skin health. Vitamin E used internally and externally will help maintain a healthy skin. Multi-minerals are essential for proper skin function. Silicon (heals skin irritations), selenium and zinc are all involved in skin healing. Potassium, manganese, calcium and magnesium are also necessary.

HERBAL COMBINATIONS—Allergy, Blood Purifiers, Bone(rich in silicon and other minerals), Digestion, Hair and Skin formulas, Immune, Liver and Gall bladder, Lower Bowels, Nerve, Potassium and Stress combinations.

SINGLE HERBS—Key herbs: Alfalfa (rich in vitamin A and minerals), Aloe Vera, Burdock, Comfrey (heals and builds cells), Dandelion, Golden Seal, Horsetail, Oatstraw, Queen of the Meadow, Red Clover, Scullcap, Yellow Dock (rich in iron). Other important herbs: Buchu (cleans kidneys), Capsicum, Chaparral (cleans blood and eliminates toxins), Cornsilk (kidney and bladder cleanser), Echinacea, Fenugreek, Gotu Kola, Hawthorn, Hops, Ho Shou-Wu, Lady's Slipper, Lobelia, Mistletoe, Pau D'Arco, Wood Betony, Wormwood.

SUPPLEMENTS—Aloe Vera juice (external and internal), Evening Primrose oil, Salmon Oil, Lecithin, Black Ointment (external for healing), Chinese essential oils, Chlorophyll, Redmond Clay (external), Tea Tree Oil (external).

AVOID—High fat and high meat diet. Alcohol, tobacco, caffeine drinks. Sugar and white flour products. Birth control pills. Some drugs cause skin problems. Avoid rancid oils, soft drinks, chocolate, potato chips and all junk food. Avoid too much salt.

STRESS

Everyone is plagued with stress. It should not be considered all bad as long as we are capable of handling situations we need to face. Stress can be beneficial and can challenge and motivate us to accomplish the seemingly impossible task. The way we choose to deal with it is the key to coping. If not controlled properly, stress can become "distress." Stressful situations can build up over the years and take a toll on our physical and emotional health. We need to strengthen our bodies so we can withstand any stress we need to. We need to learn to avoid stress we cannot handle and to handle stress we cannot avoid. Some ways to do this is by nutritionally building our nerves, fortifying our immune system, and learning to relax and exercise.

Stress can accumulate in the body and eventually cause a break down of the adrenal glands. This will cause exhaustion and a complete weakening of the emotional and physical body. It may take twenty years to accomplish this, but it will happen if long-term stress is allowed to continue. It could be a high-pressure job that you are not happy with, or a bad marriage, unresolved financial problems, loneliness. It could be a death in the family. I see couples suffer who have no children, and I also see couples who have children suffer. It isn't the situation you are in, it's how you cope with your life situations.

When the body is completely burned out because of nutrient lack, stress can control life's situation. The body, especially the nerves, have to be nourished and fed. Sugar is one of the worst things you can put in the body that will wear it down and cause exhaustion. Sugar depletes nutrients from the system. Yet we use sugar to give us a life, only to have the adrenals eventually burn out.

Symptoms of adrenal exhaustion are: Chronic Fatigue, Irritability, Health problems, Anxiety, Depression, Low Stress Tolerance, the feeling of being unable to cope or stay in touch with reality, Nervous Exhaustion, Insomnia, Difficulty in relaxing, and Panic attacks.

NATURAL THERAPY—Relaxation therapy is an art to learn. It is possible for anyone to use and benefit from it. Blood Purification, and Lower Bowel Cleansing. This will keep the blood clean so that toxins cannot travel to the brain and nerves and cause stress. A nutritional diet is necessary. A change of diet is the first step in conquering stress.

FOODS TO HEAL—The following foods are rich in vitamin A, calcium, and vitamin C: Carrots and carrot juice, yams, kale, parsley, turnip greens, collard greens, swiss chard, watercress, red and green peppers, winter squash, egg yolk, endive, persimmons, apricots and cantaloupe, broccoli, leaf lettuce, peaches, cherries, Strawberries, oranges, grapefruit, cantaloupe, green onions, limes, tangerines, tomatoes, raspberries. Foods high in magnesium and other essential minerals are: Blackstrap molasses, sunflower seeds, whole grains, almonds, soybeans, pecans, hazelnuts, oats, brown rice, Millet, white and red beans, wild rice, rye, beet greens, lentils, dried figs, lima beans, apricots, dried, dates, peaches, okra, parsley.

VITAMINS AND MINERALS—Vitamin A promotes growth and repair of body tissues. It is used up quickly when a person is under stress. B-complex are known as the "stress vitamins". They fortify the nervous system. Many people will not take B-vitamins because they say it makes them sick. The reason it causes nausea or disruptions is the liver is adjusting to having nutrients it needs and it will take time for it to adjust to good nutrition. The liver is also filtering out toxins. Folic Acid aids in the assimilation of pantothenic acid. PABA is needed to aid in the production of pantothenic acid. Vitamin C stimulates adrenal function and protects vitamin E, calcium, hormones, and enzymes from destruction. Vitamin E protects the glands when under stress.

Take a multi-mineral supplement with extra calcium for the nerves, potassium aids in insomnia; Magnesium calms the nerves. An iron deficiency causes fatigue; selenium for immune protection; Zinc nourishes the thymus gland, it is destroyed under stress.

HERBAL COMBINATIONS—Blood Purifier, Immune, Lower Bowel, Nerve and Stress formulas.

SINGLE HERBS—Key herbs: Alfalfa, Chamomile, Ginkgo (strengthens the brain), Gotu Kola (brain food), Hops, Kelp, Lady's Slipper, Licorice, Lobelia, Mistletoe, Mullein, Passion Flower, Pau D'Arco, Rose Hips (rich in B-vitamins), Scullcap (improves nerves), Suma (builds immunity), Valerian, Wood Betony.

SUPPLEMENTS—Bee Pollen, Evening Primrose Oil, Salmon Oil, Lecithin (feeds the nerves), Blue-green algae. Acidophilus, Chlorophyll (clean the blood).

AVOID—Tranquilizers. They eventually cause more stress than they alleviate. All drugs cause a stress on the body. Over-the-counter drugs deplete the body of nutrients to protect against stress. White sugar products, and white flour products. Rancid oils, fried foods. Alcohol, tobacco and caffeine will all deplete the body and cause stress.

STROKES

(natural remedies for prevention)

Many health oriented doctors, who have treated thousands of people suffering from stroke, feel that most strokes can be prevented. A stroke is a loss of functioning brain tissue, either temporary or permanent.

There are two kinds of strokes. One type is cerebral hemorrhage where a weak place in a blood vessel in the brain gives way. It is most likely to happen to those with high blood pressure. It can also happen to those with clogged and weak arteries. The second kind is cerebral thrombosis, and is due to a clot or other blockage (arteriosclerosis) in the blood vessel in the brain.

A mild attack can cause temporary confusion and lightheadedness, difficulty in speaking clearly, weakness on one side of the body, vision dimness, and confusion, severe speech difficulties, sudden or gradual loss or blurring of consciousness. Amnesia can also occur, which is often not permanent. A coma can result for short or long periods.

Some early warnings of stroke may include one or more of the following. They may only last for a few moments: fainting, stumbling, numbness or paralysis of the fingers of one hand, blurring of vision, seeing bright lights, loss of speech or memory. It is much wiser and less expensive to prevent this crippling disease and start on improving health.

A poisoned blood stream sets the stage for a possible stroke. The blood containing poisons is flowing through the arterial system, nearly a thousand miles of arteries and veins, besides many more thousand miles of capillaries. The walls of the arteries consist of cells which are subject to the same injury from toxins as the cells in the kidneys. The kidneys degenerate at the same time as do the arteries and from the same causes. When the walls thicken and harden this causes degeneration. As they harden they become more brittle, and easier to burst under pressure.

The brain has delicate blood vessels, and as the hole through the arteries grows smaller and the pressure increases and as the walls become more brittle, extra pressure causes a blood vessel to rupture, which causes a stroke. The brain cells rely on oxygen-rich blood for nourishment. If they don't receive this nourishment the brain cells die.

NATURAL THERAPY—Blood Purification, Stimulation Therapy, Lower Bowel Cleansing. A natural oral chelation will clean the entire system and help the blood flow freely. It will improve circulation so that proper nutrition and oxygen can reach the brain. Short fasting and a change of diet will also help to clean the arteries.

Eating less and more nutritious food will help heal and restore the health of the veins. High blood pressure severely strains the arteries, and if the arteries have cholesterol plaques, it can set the body up for a stroke.

Stress is a big contributor of strokes. Yet stress is hard to determine. A person isn't usually aware they are under stress. Someone who is always angry, or hateful have an extra excretion of hormones and acids, raising blood pressure, thus contributing to strokes or heart disease.

FOODS TO HEAL—High fiber foods such as whole grains: oats, wheat, barley, millet, buckwheat (contains rutin which strengthens the veins, cornmeal. Brown rice, wild rice, beans, nuts, seeds (sesame seeds contain nutrients for capillary health). Vegetables are rich in minerals and low in calories. Potatoes (baked), carrots, celery, cauliflower, cabbage, beets, onions, cucumbers, green peppers. Use vegetable salads with leaf lettuce, tomatoes, greens. String beans, snow peas, sweet potatoes.Onions, garlic, scallions, ginger, cayenne pepper have anti-clotting effect.

VITAMINS AND MINERALS—Vitamins A and E are antioxidants, bringing more oxygen to the blood, and act as free radical scavengers. Vitamin E is essential for supplying oxygen to the heart muscles. Vitamin C with bioflavonoids protects the capillaries and cleans and strengthens the veins. The B-complex vitamins improves all-over good health. They improve liver function, feed the nerves and brain and help clean and feed the veins.

Minerals are essential for pure blood and to keep the body's chemistry in balance. Minerals are essential for blood circulation. Iron is essential to supply oxygen to the cells. Selenium and zinc protect the immune system. Silicon helps the body utilize calcium and prevent it from adhering to the veins. Potassium is necessary for a healthy heart. Calcium and magnesium are needed for nerves and brain. Stress is one cause of strokes, and vitamins and minerals help fortify the nerves and brain.

HERBAL COMBINATIONS—Heart and Blood Pressure formulas, Glands, Nerves, Bone, Chelation, Digestion, Potassium.

SINGLE HERBS—Key herbs: Capsicum (cleans veins, strengthens the walls of the arteries), Bugleweed (alleviates pain in heart), Burdock, Butcher's Broom (improves circulation), Ephedra, Garlic, Ginkgo (improves mental clarity), Gotu Kola (feeds the brain), Hawthorn, Hops, Horsetail, Kelp, Passion Flower, Parsley, Pau D'Arco, Psyllium, Rose Hips, Saffron, Scullcap, Valerian. Other important herbs: Alfalfa (rich in minerals), Black Cohosh (for slow pulse rate), Blessed Thistle, Dandelion, Ginseng, Lily of the Valley, Lobelia, Yellow Dock.

SUPPLEMENTS—Chlorophyll (rebuilds heart), Lecithin (prevent fatty deposits), Flaxseed, Evening Primrose Oil, Salmon Oil, Glucomannan, Rice Bran Syrup, CoQ10, Germanium.

AVOID—Constipation (throws toxins into the bloodstream which weaken the blood vessels). Avoid smoking, alcohol, drugs of all kinds. Chlorinated water can weaken the veins. High fat and meat diet weaken the veins. Avoid too many dairy products.

Avoid stress like the plague, change to a more relaxing life-style. Enjoy life, become a more forgiving person, and learn to love and appreciate those around you.

TICKS, LICE, BED BUGS, FLEAS

(Lyme Disease, Rocky Mountain Spotted Fever)

Hahnemann, the father of homeopathy, recognized the hereditary transmission of disease (where a baby can inherit whatever her parents or ancestors have passed on), and proclaimed it in his theory of psora (an itching disease of the skin). He taught that the ordinary itch eruptions (scabies) are accompanied by the elimination of internal scrofulous infestations, which in turn, are a survival of the ancient leprosy. He asserted that systematic suppression of the external lepra continued throughout the ages, gradually transformed this external skin disease into the internal psora (skin disease) which manifests occasionally on the surface in the acute forms of itch, lice, crab-lice, hives, itchy eczemata, etc., and internally, as tuberculosis, cancer, sarcoma, asthma and other chronic destructive diseases.

Ticks, lice, bed bugs and fleas cannot live in a clean body.

Not everyone is infested with them, but those whose internal and external conditions supply the little varmints with food to support their life. When the body is cleaned and purified, when the blood is pure the lice and etc. leave.

Head lice are most often found on the scalp and hair, behind the ears and the back of the neck. The tiny nits (eggs) are laid at the base of a hair shaft; the attached egg moves away from the scalp as the hair grow. Itching is one symptom; another is when you can see the lice and eggs, which may look like dandruff.

Crab lice are transmitted mainly by sexual contact and are found in the genital areas. They can be transmitted by using a toilet seat where infestation is present. Itching is a symptom as well as the appearance of tiny black dots clinging to the base of the hairs. The lice can spread to the eyelashes, beard or hair on the chest.

Many people feel that lice are a sign of uncleanliness. It is but not meaning that you live in filth. It means that the body has either inherited weakness or have acquired toxins that contribute to these infestations. White sugar in the body contributes to these bugs.

Tick bites can cause Rocky Mountain Spotted Fever and Lyme Disease. An epidemic of these ticks have been seen in some areas. Children should be inspected after playing outside in wooded, brushy areas. Especially in late spring and summer. Prevention is the best weapon. Ticks can be seen before they do their dangerous job. It takes several minutes for them to drill into the skin so inspecting yourselves and children are the best prevention.

NATURAL THERAPY—Blood Purifying and Lower Bowel cleansing to prevent toxins from staying in the blood. All bugs, parasite and lice, bed bugs, etc., live on the toxins that have accumulated in the body from what we call autointoxication. Dr. Henry Lindlhar, used diet, and cold water treatment and a comb to get rid of lice and other bugs. He said that treating them with antiseptics and strong drugs would only push them further into the body and especially in the head area and cause headaches, dizziness, loss of memory, deafness and weakness of sight.

To remove ticks that have imbedded into the body, first pour alcohol, or olive oil to smother the tick and than carefully twist the tick with a pair of tweezers and gently pull. If the head is left in it could cause infections. I have removed many of these from my children's bodies, and we were lucky not to get infected.

With body lice, bed bugs, and any varmint the clothing should be sterilized. They live only on the body when they want to feed. Soak combs and brushes in Lysol with hot water for about thirty minutes. Freezing will also kill bugs. A solution of vinegar, lemon juice and olive oil can be applied at night or a couple of hours and than shampooed. Try to use natural methods to prevent pushing them further in the body for problems later on.

For the hair and other areas make a solution of golden seal, black walnut and aloe vera juice and put it on the area for about an hour, than shampoo or wipe off.

FOODS TO HEAL—Fruit is cleansing for the body. Use organic fruit if possible. Bugs cannot live in a clean body. Wheatgrass juice is very beneficial to cleanse and nourish the blood. Green drinks using, pure apple juice or pineapple juice with sprouts, spinach, comfrey, and parsley or any green leafy vegetables. Sulphur vegetables will help kill the eggs and bugs. Horseradish, kale, cabbage, brussels sprouts, cauliflower, chervil and watercress.

Other foods high in sulphur are cranberry, turnip, spinach, savoy cabbage, red cabbage, parsnip, leek, onions, garlic, kohlrabi, radishes, okra, swiss chard, chives. Pumpkin seeds (grind and put on food every day).

VITAMINS AND MINERALS—A clean body is essential inside and outside. Vitamins and minerals help keep the body clean. Vitamin A, heals the mucus membranes and protects the immune system. B-complex vitamins protect the nerves. C with bioflavonoids help protect the cells and immune system. Vitamin E supplies oxygen to the cells. Multi-minerals are vital. Calcium and magnesium, sulphur, selenium, and zinc protect the body. Selenium, vitamin A, and E are antioxidant and free radical scavenger (protects the cells).

HERBAL COMBINATIONS—Blood Purifiers, Digestion, Immune, Liver, Lower Bowel formulas, Parasites formulas and Potassium.

SINGLE HERBS—Key herbs: Black Walnut (kills parasites & worms), Burdock (cleans blood), Chaparral (purifies blood), Garlic, Golden Seal, Horsetail, Kelp, Pau D'Arco, Psyllium, Red Clover, Senna, Wormwood, Yellow Dock. Other beneficial herbs: Alfalfa, Aloe Vera, Buchu, Cornsilk, Echinacea, Hops, Gotu Kola, Lobelia, Papaya, Parsley, Peppermint, St. Johnswort, Uva Ursi, Wood Betany, Yarrow.

SUPPLEMENTS—Chlorophyll, Bentonite, Diatomaceous Earth, Garlic extract, Glucomannan, Spirulina.

AVOID—All junk food, fried food, white sugar and white flour products. Pastry, cookies, candy, ice cream. Avoid meat, even chicken can harbor bugs. Use a natural insect repellent to avoid ticks and other bugs.

TONSILLITIS AND STREP THROAT

Tonsillitis does not necessarily mean there is a strep infection. But tonsillitis, sore throat, swollen glands in the neck, sinusitis, and middle ear infections could mean a streptococcus infection is present. The strep germ can do much harm and indirectly cause rheumatic fever and nephritis (kidney disease).

When a child does not seem to be recovering from a cold, sore throat or bronchial infection, or a fever develops when a cold seems to be subsiding may suggest a potential serious complication. Also, if fever headaches and vomiting continue and the throat becomes so sore that it is hard to swallow a health doctor should be consulted.

The tonsils are one of the body's protections against airborne bacteria entering the system through the mouth and nose. These work with the lymphatic system to fight infections. The tonsils are a protection, and when they become inflamed it is nature's way of telling you to clean out the body. When sore throats are constantly irritated with drugs (which suppress the acute disease), overeating and lack of rest, the mucus that is trying to eliminate is thrown back into the system to cause a worse problem next time. If the tonsils continue to become inflamed it will eventually accumulate scar tissue and prevent the tonsils from doing what nature intended. If you have lost both your tonsils and appendix through surgery, an extra burden is put on the lymphatics.

NATURAL THERAPY—Blood Purification and Lower Bowel Cleansing are needed. A three day juice fast will help nature heal. Use citrus juices, herbal teas, herbal extracts, chiropractic, foot reflexology and massage therapy for improved circulation. The body needs to throw off the mucus that is overloading the system. If you eat during nature's cleanse (acute diseases are nature's way of cleansing and healing the body), the body has to stop cleansing and digest food, which puts toxins further into the body, to emerge as a chronic disease later.

Bed rest and relaxation are necessary for the body to heal itself. This means relaxation in the mind as well as the body.

Enemas, colonics or herbal bowel cleansers will speed the healing process. This will bring the fever down in a natural way.

FOODS TO HEAL—Citrus juices, oranges, lemons, limes and grapefruit will cleanse the lymphatics. Herbal teas help nature clean and eliminate the toxins. Pure water and herbal teas flush out the toxins that the cells squeeze into the stomach.

VITAMINS AND MINERALS—Vitamin A (high amounts at first). Vitamin C with bioflavonoids will heal and flush out the toxins. Vitamin B-complex vitamins are needed to rebuild after acute disease is passed. They are depleted fast in illness. Multi-mineral with extra calcium and magnesium (in herbal form), potassium, selenium, silicon and zinc.

HERBAL COMBINATIONS—Blood Purifier, Allergy formulas, Cold and Flu formulas, Infection, Lower Bowel, Nerve and Potassium formulas.

SINGLE HERBS—Key Herbs: Alfalfa and mint tea, Aloe Vera (laxative and attracts toxins to be eliminated), Fenugreek and Comfrey together (break up mucus), Echinacea (a special herb to help clean the lymphatics), Ginger (settles stomach), Golden Seal (a strong antibiotic), Kelp (will clean and nourish), Lobelia (the greatest healer of the stomach, which is the center of disease), Marshmallow (healing to the mucus membranes), Passion Flower, Hops, Scullcap (and all nervine herbs will relax the body for nature to heal), Red Raspberry (in tea form for fast assimilation), Pau D'Arco (protects the liver and cleans the blood), Rose Hips (rich in vitamin C and B-complex vitamins), Slippery Elm (for coughs and heals the throat and stomach), also contains protein for healing and building the cells).

SUPPLEMENTS—Green drinks, Chlorophyll, Lemon-lime drinks mixed with herbal extracts. Rice bran syrup, essential fatty acids, Evening Primrose Oil, Salmon Oil. Chinese essential oil,(rub on throat and neck to help pain).

AVOID—Stop eating during an acute disease. Avoid caffeine, alcohol, tobacco, and over the counter drugs. They will only suppress the elimination. Avoid sugar and white flour products.

ULCERS

Ulcers are one of the plagues of modern day living. It has been well established that emotional stress and anxiety are one of the main causes of gastric ulcers. The pit of the stomach is often used as a sounding board for our emotions. Nine out of ten people who acquire ulcers get them through fretting, worrying over existing, or non-existing problems in life. It seems that in order to prevent gastric ulcers there is a need to find ways to handle life's problems that will not effect the stomach. There has to be a way to combat tensions that will prevent the stomach from suffering.

Autointoxication and constipation are other causes of ulcers. When the lower colon is clogged and delays the passage of food from the system, fermentation and acid conditions which irritate the stomach wall will result. During acute disease the cells have to squeeze toxins and dump them in the stomach to be removed from the body through the colon. When diseases are suppressed with drugs or eating, it stops the cleansing and the stomach becomes irritated. When this is done often it weakens the stomach muscles.

An ulcer simply means an open sore. Peptic ulcers indicate that the sore is in the stomach or the duodenum, the first part of the intestines which connect with the stomach. It is associated with the presence of an excessive amount of acid gastric juice. This is the digestive juice that is necessary for digestion. Worry and anxiety increase the secretion of the stomach. You should never eat when you are worried or feel anxious.

The most common symptom of an ulcer is a burning sensation or discomfort in the upper abdomen, usually felt about two or three hours after meals or in the middle of the night. Nausea and vomiting may occur. Sometimes an ulcer will cause bleeding, and a slow seeping of blood may cause anemia.

NATURAL THERAPY—Tranquilization therapy using nervine herbs to strengthen the nervous system. The stomach feels every emotion you have and needs to be healed. With stomach ulcers, a person's vitality and strength are weakened and they need help to repair and heal. If constipation is the problem, enemas and juice fasts can help. Freshly squeezed cabbage juice will heal ulcers. Aloe Vera juice is healing, it inhibits the secretion of hydrochloric acid.

Proper chewing is essential. Proper food combining is vital to give the stomach time for healing and restoring vitality. Doctors used to recommend bland diets, but find that they are not beneficial. They contain no nourishment.

FOODS TO HEAL—Slippery Elm is an herb, which is considered a food that will heal ulcers and provide protein and nourishment as well. Potatoes are healing; they have an alkaline reaction and help neutralize acid production. Bake them at 500 degrees, this changes them from a starch to glucose. Almonds, well-chewed, will heal and do not cause an over-production of acid. Almond milk helps to neutralize excess acid in the stomach. Carrots and carrot juice will heal and are very high in calcium and vitamin A. Millet, brown rice, buckwheat and yellow corn meal will heal, but need to be cooked slowly in a thermos to retain enzymes. Rejuvelac is a healthy enzyme drink. It acts as a protection against harmful organisms in the intestinal tract. It is rich in protein, carbohydrates, B-complex vitamins as well as vitamins E and K. (K protects against bleeding). The recipe for thermos cooking is in my Today's Healthy Eating book.

Barley helps to rebuild the lining of the stomach and soothes ulcers with its rich content of B1 and B2, and bioflavonoids. Cook slowly in a thermos to retain the B-vitamins.

Okra powder acts as a demulcent to stop inflammation. Eat papaya often. It contains enzymes to improve digestion and is very healing to the stomach lining. Persimmons, an energy food, also heals and soothes the mucus membranes of the stomach. Sprouts contain live enzymes, protein, vitamins and minerals. Sweet potatoes are soothing and nourishing. Whey powder contains natural sodium that is healing to ulcers.

VITAMINS AND MINERALS—Vitamin A protects the stomach acid from irritation. Vitamins A and E together form a protection against ulcers developing, as well as heal. Vitamin C with bioflavonoids will heal ulcers. Vitamin E will also heal scar tissues. (Remember all sores cause scar tissue to form). Minerals are important in healing ulcers. Iron builds rich blood and helps restore vitality. Vitamin K prevents bleeding. Calcium and magnesium heal the nerves and help in ulcers. Potassium helps balance excess acid. Selenium, silicon and zinc help heal ulcers.

HERBAL COMBINATIONS—Blood Purifiers, Bone (rich in minerals), Comfrey and Pepsin, Digestion, Lower Bowels, Nerve and Ulcer formulas.

SINGLE HERBS—Key herbs: Alfalfa (rich in minerals an vitamins, especially K), Aloe Vera, Capsicum, Comfrey, Fenugreek, Garlic, Golden Seal (very healing for the digestive system), Hops (for the nerves), Kelp, Lady's Slipper, Lobelia, Oatstraw, Pau D'Arco, Psyllium, Scullcap, Slippery Elm, White Oak. Other important herbs are: Black Walnut, Burdock, Dandelion, Echinacea, Ginger, Hawthorn, Myrrh, Watercress, Yellow Dock (rich in iron).

SUPPLEMENTS—Aloe Vera Juice, Liquid Chlorophyll, Glucomannan, Evening Primrose Oil, Salmon Oil, Blue-green algae. Bee Pollen helps heal digestive system. Flaxseed tea coats the digestive tract and protects the sores. (Simmer two tablespoons in a pint of water for about three or four minutes. Propolis heals ulcers and contains antibiotic properties.

AVOID—Heated vegetable oil may cause ulcers. Don't eat when under stress. Antacids can upset the metabolic balance of the body. Cimetidine is widely prescribed for the pain but does not cure the ulcers. It could cause cancer, and even sterility. Aspirin can cause bleeding and ulcers. Smoking inhibits pancreatic bicarbonate secretion and can cause ulcers. Food stagnation can cause ulcers. Avoid white sugar and flour; they stimulate acid production.

Bibliography

Austin, Phylis, Agatha Thrash, M.D. and Calvin Thrash, M.D., M.P.H., Natural Healthcare For Your Child, 1990. Natural Remedies, 1983, Published by Family Health Publication, Sunfield, Mich.

Balch, James F., M.D. and Balch, Phyllis A. C.N.C., 1990. Published by Avery Publishing Group, Inc., Garden City Park, New York.

Baroody, Theodore A., Jr., M.A., D.C., 1987. Published by OMNI Learning Institute, Asheville, N.C.

Cayetano, H.J.M., Building Vital Health, 1988. Published by The Eastern Publishing Association, Manila.

Douglass, William Campbell, M.D. Aids The End of Civilization, 1989. Published by Valet Publishers, Clayton, Georgia.

Galland, Leo, M.D., with Dian Dincin Buchaman, Ph.D. Superimmunity for Kids. 1988. Published by Delta Book, New York, N.Y.

Hoffman, David, The Holistic Herbal, 1983. Published by The Findhorn Press, Scotland.

James, Walene, Immunization The Reality Behind The Myth, 1988. Published by Gergen & Gravey Publishers, Inc., Massachusetts.

Fox, William, M.D., Family Botanic Guide or Every Man His Own Doctor, 1904.

Lindlahr, Henry, M.D., Natural Therapeutics, Vol. 1, 2 and 6. Philosophy of Natural Therapeutics, 1918. Practice of Natural Therapeutics, 1919. Iridiagnosis and other Diagnostic Methods, 1922.

Mudd, Chris, Cholesterol and Your Health, The Great American Rip Off. Published by American Lite Co., Oklahoma City, OK.

Pierce, R.V., M.D., The Peoples Common Sense Medical Adviser, 1895.

Roberts, Frank, Modern Herbalism for Digestive Disorders, 1978. Published by Thorsons Publishing Limited, England.

Lust, John, N.D. and Michael Tierra, C.A., O.M.D. The Natural Remedy Bible. Published by Pocket Book, Simon and Schuster, 1990.

ad, Dr. Vasant and Frawley, David, The Yoga of Herbs, 1986. Published by Lotus Press, Santa Fe, New Mexico.

LePore, Donald, N.D., The Ultimate Healing System, 1985. Published by Woodland Books, Provo, Utah.

Muramoto, Noboru, Natural Immunity, Insights on Diet and Aids. 1988. Published by George Ohsawa Macrobiotic Foundation, Oroville, California.

Stevens, Dr. John, Medical Reform or Physiology and Botanic Practice, London, 1847.

Santilli, Humbart, B.S., M.H. Natural Healing with Herbs, 1984. Published by Hohm Press, Prescott Valley, AZ.

Scott, Julian, Ph.D. Natural Medicine for Children, 1990. Published by Avon Books, New York, N.Y.

Stone, Dr. Randolph, D.O., D.C., 1985. Published by CRCS Published, Sebastopol, California.

Tenney, Louise M.H. Today's Herbal Health, Today's Healthy Eating, Modern Day Plagues and Health Handbook. Published by Woodland Books, Provo, Utah.

Thomson, Samuel, 1835. New Guide To Health or Botanic Family Physician.

Tierra, Michael, C.A., N.D., The Way of Herbs, 1980. Published by Unity Press, Santa Cruz, California. Planetary Herbology, 1988. Published by Lotus Press, Santa Fe, New Mexico.

Theiss, Barbara and Peter, The Family Herbal, 1989. Published by Healing Arts Press, Rochester, Vermont.

Truss, C. Orian, M.D. The Missing Diagnosis, 1983. Published by The Missing Diagnosis, Inc., Birmingham, Alabama.

Weiss, Rudolf, Fritz, M.D., Herbal Medicine, 1988. Distributed by Medicina Biologica, Portland, Oregon.

Welles, William F., D.C., The Shocking Truth About Cholesterol, 1990. Published by William F. Welles, D.C.

Willard, Terry, Ph.D., Helping Yourself with Natural Remedies, 1951. Published by CRCS Publications, Reno, Nevada.

Index